REPRODUCTIVE RIGHTS AS HUMAN RIGHTS

Reproductive Rights as Human Rights

Women of Color and the Fight for Reproductive Justice

Zakiya Luna

NEW YORK UNIVERSITY PRESS

New York

NEW YORK UNIVERSITY PRESS
New York
www.nyupress.org

Parts of Chapter 5 initially appeared from the following published article: "Marching Toward Reproductive Justice: Coalition (Re)Framing of the March for Women's Lives," *Sociological Inquiry* (2010). Used with permission.

References to Internet websites (URLs) were accurate at the time of writing. Neither the author nor New York University Press is responsible for URLs that may have expired or changed since the manuscript was prepared.

Please contact the Library of Congress for Cataloging-in-Publication data.

ISBN: 978-1-4798-5202-4 (hardback)
ISBN: 978-1-4798-3129-6 (paperback)

New York University Press books are printed on acid-free paper, and their binding materials are chosen for strength and durability. We strive to use environmentally responsible suppliers and materials to the greatest extent possible in publishing our books.
Manufactured in the United States of America
10 9 8 7 6 5 4 3 2 1
Also available as an ebook

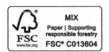

MIX
Paper | Supporting
responsible forestry
FSC
www.fsc.org FSC® C013604

To mom: Thanks for bringing us to anti-apartheid rallies, university classes, and skate rinks.

CONTENTS

Introduction

While it was a warm and humid day in Miami, Florida that July day in 2011, the air conditioning blasted inside the hotel lobby. Low lights were on although they seemed almost unnecessary with the sun illuminating the space. Low music filled the air, almost covered by the clatter of people talking in a variety of languages. Further back, a curving staircase spanned the back of the lobby—it would become the setting for various conference photos, including a "Black reproductive justice" one in which Black women, including myself, posed to show the legacy of Black women in reproductive justice activism.[1] The bottom stair ended near the floor-to-ceiling windows, which highlighted the main attraction that awaited guests: a deck with poolside service. Behind the deck, a wooden boardwalk went on for miles, followed by a dreamy expanse of beach that cuddled the sapphire ocean as far as the eye could see. To the right of the entrance, the slick white floor tile led to the official conference ballroom that would serve as the site for the plenaries for SisterSong Women of Color Reproductive Justice Collective's "Let's Talk about Sex!" (LTAS) conference.

At the time, SisterSong was—and to some extent still is—the group most associated with the phrase "reproductive justice" (RJ) and its basic definition: the right to not have children, the right to have children, and the right to parent.[2] Thus, SisterSong gatherings attracted an array of participants experienced in organizations for reproductive health, reproductive rights, and reproductive justice, or just interested generally. Throughout the following days, hundreds of conference attendees—women, men, and gender-nonbinary people—would pass through that lobby. They would wear everything from African dashikis to peasant blouses to skin-tight leather, with shoes ranging from Converse sneakers to high heels. Attendees wore their hair in cropped cuts, braids, and Afros, in a range of colors, some of which matched Miami's fauna, and some were even bald. They were of various racial backgrounds and skin tones. Laughter, yelps, and multiple languages filled the air throughout the day. Some lived in Miami whereas others had traveled across the globe for the momentous event.

This was the first LTAS conference since 2007, and since the election of President Obama. The 2011 theme was "Love, Legislation, Leadership." The organizers chose the beach location purposefully: "We intentionally planned this weekend as a 'destination conference' because we know how much Reproductive Justice activists work. It is non-stop and often we do not allow time to take care of ourselves."[3] The opening plenary began with a "Welcome to the Indigenous Land" by two women from area tribes. The conference coordinators welcomed us, followed by a city commissioner who awkwardly encouraged us to talk about sex "but not on the boardwalk," reminding us of the appropriate social norms. During the opening plenary, SisterSong's national coordinator, Loretta Ross, welcomed everyone. LTAS 2011 was an even more special conference than most, as Ross announced that she was retiring after over a decade with the collective; Laura Jiménez, the long-time deputy coordinator, would leave SisterSong to direct California Latinas for Reproductive Justice; and Heidi Williamson, the policy coordinator, was leaving to work in Washington, DC. As Ross gave the history of SisterSong, she proclaimed, "RJ exists because of human rights."

Over those days, about fifty workshops occurred. Preconference institutes had already included SisterSong staff presenting RJ101 and RJ102, Hampshire College's Civil Liberties and Public Policy Institute for young leaders of color, a Queer People of Color and Indigenous People (QPOC) institute hosted by SisterSong's QPOC mini-community, and another on White women as allies. Dorothy Roberts signed books in an upstairs room, where organizations and vendors staffed tables. Brown Girl Burlesque (BGB) performed one evening, which garnered some controversy. When the idea of BGB performing had been raised earlier in the year, the idea received both support and opposition from key people in SisterSong, who held different views on the place of the erotic in women of color's self-expression. To bring the conversation to a larger set of people, SisterSong had hosted a public conference call a few months prior in which the focus was the politics of sex work.[4] At LTAS, the BGB performance was highly promoted, as was BGB's preceding conference workshop. The workshop offered an opportunity to meet the performers and learn about their philosophy of burlesque as an empowering practice for women of color. Fliers and word of mouth advertised other events—for example, that the cervical self-exam workshop would occur in a private hotel room rather than a standard conference room.

Throughout those few days people shared their experiences in the movements for reproductive health, rights, and justice, laughed, danced, reveled in nature—including a group who went skinny dipping in the warm water at night—learned from each other, and just breathed. These few days were ones of joyous community as the reproductive justice movement subtly modeled the goal: to make life always feel like this. It was a reminder that human flourishing meant not just mere existence, but people being able to express their full humanity and have that humanity respected and even celebrated by the people around them. We understood that this was what it could feel like if SisterSong realized its mission: "to amplify and strengthen the collective voices of Indigenous women and women of color to ensure reproductive justice *through securing human rights*."[5]

In this book I explore in more depth what this mission meant. When defining the US reproductive justice movement, various activists and scholars note that reproductive justice is "human rights–based." In many scholarly and activist accounts, the phrases "human rights" and "reproductive justice" are continually linked, as if there was an inevitability to the way the RJ movement developed. Yet, the way "human rights" has been conceptualized and received in movement practice has not been clarified.

Reproductive Rights as Human Rights highlights an underexamined mobilization strategy within the US context and reveals both the promise and the problems associated with a human rights approach. Furthermore, given SisterSong's status as a coalition led by and focused on women of color and their reproductive rights, the book brings a much-needed intersectional lens to bear on social movements operating in an increasingly globalized context. I draw on interviews, observations, and archival documents collected over four years of fieldwork and research to trace the way SisterSong balanced a commitment to human rights with the reality of a government hostile to enforcing expansive human rights standards within its own country. In addition, I show how activists engaged with and sought to educate a public—including fellow activists in their own and other movements—largely uninformed about human rights. Throughout the book, I focus on human rights as norms, or ideals for treatment of other people. The tools to reinforce these norms include laws, grassroots organizing, and institution building. Community organizing does not always produce laws or institutions, but it can. The state can support, enforce, or violate human rights. Still, I, and others, argue that human rights do not reside solely in the state and instead are a relational practice.

From its founding in 1997 to the time when I completed my initial data collection, SisterSong grew to be the largest and most visible organizational coalition in the reproductive justice movement. Founded as a "project" of sixteen minority-focused women's health organizations, SisterSong held a central role in the RJ movement and continues to be one of the organizations most frequently cited in definitions of "reproductive justice" in the United States. Given widespread assumptions in the United States that human rights are relevant only in "international" contexts, SisterSong emphasizing human rights seemed an unlikely way to advance movement claims in the United States.

I argue that part of SisterSong's strategy was rooted in its *domestication of human rights*. I use the term "domestication" to describe the discursive process of relating international rhetoric to a domestic problem, and argue that this process was conducted in two very different ways by the US government and SisterSong, respectively. On the one hand, the government engaged in *restrictive domestication* of human rights, in which the US government has constrained the meaning of "human rights" to suit its domestic and international needs. It domesticated human rights by relying on narratives of exceptionalism regarding human rights—in this case, a strategy of containing the definition and scope of human rights domestically, so they appear to be lacking only in *other* countries. This watered-down version of rights develops through a focus on only certain types of human rights—namely, civil and political rights—at the expense of others. The restrictive mode of domestication connotes taming and containment. In contrast, SisterSong engaged in what I call *revolutionary domestication* of human rights, in which it insisted on the relevance of internationally recognized human rights in the domestic political arena of the United States, and highlighted precisely the kind of social and economic factors shaping access to rights that restrictive domestication sought to obscure. This strategy essentially turned the state's domestication strategy on its head by actively working to bring international human rights "home," so to speak, and insisting on their relevance and need to be protected within the United States. Revolutionary domestication constructs international human rights discourse as relevant and necessary for the domestic political sphere while challenging the public (state) and private (domestic) binary.

I argue that from its start, SisterSong continually linked reproductive politics and human rights, albeit inconsistently. Framing its grievances in terms of "reproductive justice" and continually shifting the primacy of the "human rights" frame enabled SisterSong founders to proffer an analysis of structural inequality and its impact on their communities' reproductive possibilities; unite SisterSong's constituents' diverse identities into a single movement; and retain a level of rhetorical flexibility when confronted with unforeseen reproductive concerns. The framework of human rights *was* radical due to being embedded in an idea that challenged the dominant US discourse—a fact SisterSong leveraged to its advantage by presenting human rights as simultaneously radical yet familiar, and better but not opposed to other popular framing options, including those of civil rights and social justice. It is precisely because human rights were so "radical" in the US context that SisterSong was able to claim for itself what scholars refer to as a niche, which provided an advantage for it as a social movement organization (SMO).[6]

However, challenges came from competing imperatives that brought women together to develop SisterSong, including the general desire to create a sustainable woman of color–led movement focused on reproduction. This would in and of itself be a major task that was pregnant with a vision for a movement that could transform the landscape of the social movement field of reproduction, while also shifting power to the people most affected by issues around which the women's movement had traditionally mobilized, such as access to abortion, contraception, and other reproductive healthcare. In practice, according to the data, there were very few issues that did not disproportionately affect minority women. This was the case because of an already unequal system of state power that was—and still is—the basis of the United States' domestic and international policy. There is no longer a time that has not been touched by capitalism, which emphasizes work productivity and labor exploitation. There is no longer a time untouched by neoliberalism and its logics of austerity, disinvestment from social services, colonial legacies, or the specter of racism. That these realities—and new ones emerging such as a new international "free" trade system—were coalescing as SisterSong was developing is important to keep in mind. One of the continual tensions with SisterSong—and the broader reproductive justice movement—is that the state is implicated in the oppression of groups. Indeed, theorists as varied as Louis Althusser and Angela Davis remind us that one of the main functions of the state is social control and oppression, whether exerted through physical force, ideology, or both.[7] Yet, activists call upon the state (through its representatives) to make changes to policies in order to remedy oppression. Thus, a tension existed: if the state was responsible for upholding human rights, on which reproductive justice was to rest, then the state would hold the power to remove those human rights.

All these motivations had to be balanced, and some outweighed others over time. Thus, there was a continual tension between human rights as motivation versus human rights as strategy.[8] Human rights discourse offers a multivocal language—in this case, the idea was simultaneously leveraged to signal, on the one hand, an *idealized commitment* to the "global" as one of the *embodied values* on which this new way of understanding reproductive politics (reproductive justice) depended and, on the other hand, a *vision* of a future. Since these different understandings existed from the early days of the collective, they remained in subtle contention in the collective's later activities, including programming and self-definition.

The history of the reproductive justice movement, and of SisterSong specifically, illustrates the complexity of many movement intersections and elisions. The movement emerged through both discord and dialogue with different wings of the women's movement and the racial justice movement, but cannot be reduced to a simple outgrowth of either.[9] The RJ movement is larger than SisterSong, but SisterSong was for decades the only national coalition of reproductive justice organizations. Furthermore, SisterSong is generally credited with popularizing the concept of "reproductive justice"; indeed, when defining the term, many people simply cite a SisterSong leader's succinct phrasing: "(1) the right to have a child; (2) the right not to have a child; and (3) the right to parent the children we have."[10]

The Atlanta-based SisterSong coalition was founded by sixteen organizations representing four different ethnic/racial groups or "mini-communities": African American, Asian/Pacific Islander, Chicano/Latino, and Indigenous/Native American. These organizations differed in size, capacity, structure, and focus, but they came together to focus on the reproductive health concerns of women of color. The Management Circle served as a board of directors. Organizational membership in the coalition has varied over the years, but at SisterSong's peak, it boasted eighty member and allied organizations—member organizations were, ideally, women of color-focused and -led. The coalition initially intended to focus on building the internal capacity of its member organizations, but expanded its reach. In 2000, an individual membership category was added, and in 2003, an Arab American mini-community was formed. Given this structure, "SisterSong" can refer to the national office in Atlanta, the entirety of the member and allied organizations, or even the individual members. Throughout the book I specify which of these I refer to since part of the book's goal is to examine the varied levels of (dis)connection with human rights.

Since SisterSong's founding, it has achieved some elements of what other scholars have defined as movement success, such as expansion of membership, increased funding, and recognition by elites. In 2003, Sister-Song held its first national conference in Atlanta, with approximately six hundred participants. Subsequent SisterSong membership meetings and conferences have all had hundreds of attendees. Through annual events such as conferences and smaller membership meetings, SisterSong provided the largest national forum for reproductive justice activists, particularly racial minority women, across a range of experience levels. Given SisterSong's longevity, many of the founders have even built relationships with liberal feminist organizations that they also challenge, such as the National Organization for Women. SisterSong's visibility with policymakers increased through a number of intentional efforts, for example, through strategizing with policy-oriented ally organizations. In 2008, First Lady Michelle Obama invited two of SisterSong's founders, Loretta Ross and Dázon Dixon Diallo, to White House discussions on healthcare reform, signaling the coalition's visibility and legitimacy. SisterSong's advocacy efforts in other realms have also received coverage in outlets such as the *New York Times*, the *Laura Ingraham Show*, and National Public Radio.

SisterSong's success, of course, like that of many SMOs, is the result of many factors, including timing, resources, and leadership. The point of this book, however, is not to identify those variables that explain SisterSong's rise in general. Rather, the book focuses on a specific strategy adopted by SisterSong and since integrated so thoroughly with the RJ movement that its history is often taken for granted—the framing of reproductive justice in terms of human rights. I locate SisterSong within the relatively sparse history of US SMOs that have championed human rights as central to their cause. What follows is not the one "true" story of a movement or even a single SMO, but rather, a story about the novelty of a movement using a human rights frame, what that use looked like in practice, and its consequences.

It is also essential to note, however, that the selection of SisterSong as my focus is far from incidental. It is not that SisterSong just "happens" to have chosen a human rights frame, thus making it an appropriate case study. Rather, as I will argue, it was precisely because of who and what SisterSong was and is—a women of color–focused and –led organization—that it adopted this specific strategy, engaging and interpreting it in particular ways. Indeed, one of the major concerns of this book is to highlight intersectional identities and their significant role in shaping movement formation and framing. The women's movement, like other social movements, is not a cleanly unified whole; its current incarnation emerges from a history of "a group of feminisms."[11] Activist and scholarly accounts are rife with tales of the damaging internal politics of the women's movement, a so-called new social movement. New social movement theory demonstrates that identity concerns are central to those social movements that do not focus solely on state-based change.[12] Identification with a movement often requires some sense of a shared identity group, concerns about injustice faced by that identity group, and commitment to working on behalf of that identity.[13] There is increasing recognition that framing processes and identity-construction processes are interrelated in many movements.[14] Previous research has suggested that collective identity is constructed primarily in response to the challenges of dominant groups external to the membership.[15] While it may seem obvious to say that frames and (collective) identity matter to movements, my point bears repeating in a society where many political leaders and the public continue to insist that the election of the nation's first Black president and multiple women having entered campaigns for president signal that we are in a "postracial" and "postfeminist" era.

Analyses by women of color have challenged the liberal strains of feminist theory and activism, which have tended to assume that the shared position of women *as* women, defined solely on the basis of gender, should take precedence over organizing against racism, classism, or homophobia. Sometimes referred to as "woman of color feminism," "multiracial feminism," "third wave feminism," or "intersectional feminism," these critiques have predominantly been made by women of color, though some White women have also supported and articulated them.[16] Becky Thompson writes of the origins of this challenge, "The women of color and White militant women who supported a race, class, and gender analysis in the late 1960s and 1970s often found themselves trying to explain their politics in mixed gender settings (at home, at work, and in their activism), sometimes alienated from the men (and some women) who did not get it, while simultaneously alienated from White feminists whose politics they considered narrow at best and frivolous at worst."[17] Dissatisfied with mainstream feminists' lack of attention to a range of issues, women of color have produced alternative frameworks to analyze inequality and to accommodate perspectives not addressed in mainstream US feminist theory and activism.

What happens when we center women of color's organizing? Or, put another way, what happens when we "bring women of color out of the footnotes"?[18] "Women of color" refers to both an identity and a political stance that, together, advance the idea that women of marginalized racial/ethnic groups experience oppression due to *both* their race and their gender, among other identities. The term "women of color" has been attributed to activists themselves. Indeed, a search engine query for "women of color definition" results in a link to a video of Loretta Ross explaining the origin of the phrase. The Wikipedia entry for "people of color" refers to the video.[19] A sociologist of gender refers to being "really excited" upon finding the video and writes about the utility of Ross's clip for explaining to students why the term is preferred to "colored people."[20] As Ross explains, in preparation for the 1977 National Women's Conference in Texas, which President Carter funded to the tune of $5 million, White conference organizers such as Eleanor Smeal wrote a three-paragraph entry titled "Minority Women's Plank" in a two-hundred-page report. To represent themselves, Black women developed a Black Women's Agenda that they aimed to have conference delegates vote to include in the final report. When women of other ethnic backgrounds learned about the agenda, they wanted to be included. Thus, the Agenda's name was changed to reflect the broader communities represented in the report.[21] While the conference's importance as the first large national convening of women is described in other places, the importance of the phrase "women of color" is not.[22]

Texts such as Moraga and Anzaldúa (1981) *This Bridge Called My Back: Writing by Radical Women of Color* provided a foundation for the recognition of a history that is composed of many racial groups but also larger than any of those individual groups. The term "women of color" has generally included Black women, Chicana/Latina women, and Asian/Pacific Islander women. Sometimes Native American women are included in the phrase, but at other times they are identified separately to indicate how, due to settler colonialism, indigenous people have a collective history of dispossession of land that continues today, as do their decolonization efforts.[23] In the past few decades, Arab American women have also come to be included in the category, and with especially renewed vigor after xenophobic responses to the September 11, 2001, attacks on the World Trade Center solidified the conflation of Arab Americans, Muslims, and terrorists. Women of color both across and within these racial/ethnic groups do not necessarily agree, just as White women do not agree on all social issues. Yet, the term suggests that while specific histories of racial marginalization in the United States produce unique experiences, these women also share commonalities around which they can connect and seek social change.[24] Drawing from both this broader history and SisterSong's specific history, *Reproductive Rights as Human Rights* foregrounds the varied voices of women of color.

Sociologists continue to write about women of color as if they were subjects who are acted upon—by their partners, by the state, or by a nebulous "society." While that *is* a part of their experience, women of color are also *active* participants in their lives and, in the context of social movements, participants who raise critical questions about the movements in which they participate or that claim to represent them. Too often, however, the activism of women of color has been subsumed under analysis that focuses on other groups. For example, in

Armstrong's influential study of gay identity, women of color, or more broadly, minorities, are presented as problem actors who will not allow the movement to proceed without continually raising the question of how race and gender (and class) will be addressed. In this way, women of color are only incorporated into the story of "the" gay community as minor and problematic players.

On the other hand, the handful of books by sociologists that have looked at organizing by minority women as the central analytic largely focus on them as members of historical movements.[25] For example, Belinda Robnett's now-lauded book *How Long? How Long? African-American Women in the Struggle for Civil Rights* focused on women's leadership and challenged the narrative (both scholarly and popular) that a small group of charismatic men guided the US civil rights movement. Benita Roth's *Separate Roads to Feminism: Black, Chicana, and White Feminist Movements in America's Second Wave* demonstrated how, rather than Black and Chicana women's activisms being derivative of White women's activism, Black and Chicana women had their own concerns and modes of organizing. While such movements are important, we know little about how women of color are engaging in more contemporary social movements. A smattering of sociological studies considers activism of Asian/Pacific Islanders, Latinos, and Native Americans, but gender is largely absent from these analyses.[26] The field is changing, but, remarkably, the subfield of social movements research has been slow to move. In fact, the first sociology journal publishing a critique of the limitations of US social movement theory to explain Black social movements was published in 2016.[27]

However, there is a long history of women of color making critical interventions in feminist and racial/ethnic movements. For example, the Boston-based Combahee River Collective articulated the difficult position in which many Black women found themselves when fighting for social justice: "We . . . often find it difficult to separate race from class from sex oppression because in our lives they are most often experienced simultaneously."[28] While the Combahee River Collective explicitly identified itself as lesbian, it rejected separatism, which was deemed an unrealistic and regressive proposition for Black women; "community" necessarily included Black men as brothers, children, and friends. Even though, legally, race and gender discrimination could not be argued for separately, in practice, different groups of women articulated a sense of multiple "jeopardy" that led to multiple experiences of discrimination that no one identity could "explain."[29]

Being a woman of a racial/ethnic minority could produce several levels of consciousness: understanding oneself as part of the collectivity of women who are in a structurally subordinate position vis-à-vis men, while simultaneously understanding oneself as part of an individual racial/ethnic group that is positioned in a structurally subordinate position vis-à-vis White people. Furthermore, there is another layer of consciousness that goes beyond understanding the need for rights for specific groups such as Asian/Pacific Islander women, Latinas, and so on: this entails recognition that membership in one subordinated racial/ethnic group provides a point of connection with other subordinated racial/ethnic groups. For activists, feelings of solidarity can result from early experiences with people from other groups, as well as imagined connections with other oppressed people.[30] Effective coalition thus requires increased analysis of one's own investments and position within global politics.[31]

Even with their emphasis on acknowledging inequality, women of color activists' scholarship and organizing supports the observation that they "generally do not subscribe to a picture of total oppression, insisting rather on the possibility and necessity of transformatory agency."[32] The questions of representation women of color posed to White women who focused solely on race-blind conceptions of gender oppression have generated conversation about feminism always needing to serve as a broader project of social transformation. Part of the appeal of a human rights framework for some women of color is precisely the potential the expansive discourse and praxis have to facilitate restructuring society while also recognizing multiple identities. Nonetheless, the decision for SisterSong to use a human rights frame was far from an obvious one for women of color dissatisfied with other movements. To understand this decision, it is necessary to understand how and why critiques by women of color clustered around questions of health and reproduction specifically.

Organizing around Women's Health and Reproduction

Historically, eugenic ideology—the belief that some populations are intrinsically superior to others and that the health of the nation depended on intervening in the reproduction of both populations—has pervaded the practices of medical authorities and state agents.[33] People of color, immigrants, people with mental disabilities, and anyone deemed "unfit" were all targets for coercive medical practices, some stories of which have been passed down among generations, resulting in continuing distrust of medical providers.[34] In turn, the argument that health is a basic right is not new, and the United States offers a rich history of activism related to this claim. Noted civil rights activist Fannie Lou Hamer was often quoted as saying she was "sick and tired of being sick and tired" and openly discussed her experience of having been forcibly sterilized.[35] Geographer Jenna Loyd points to how disparate groups of Los Angeles–area community members simultaneously fought against militarization while demanding government investment in community health programs.[36] Sociologist Alondra Nelson details how the Black Panthers fought for community-controlled health centers and against racist assumptions of medical authorities.[37] And historian Jennifer Nelson has demonstrated how feminist women's health advocates understood their activism as extending beyond medical care to include intertwined social issues.[38]

Yet US sociologists' relatively recent turn towards human rights analysis has largely focused on issues such as housing and incarceration, with little attention to health. Unsurprisingly, within that subfield, reproduction receives even less attention, despite being a site of political controversy in the United States. For example, a number of edited volumes appeared that include examples of activism in the United States that could be considered human rights organizing. Shareen Hertel and Kathryn Libal's *Human Rights in the United States: Beyond Exceptionalism* considered a range of social problems and offered readers examples of how these issues could be examined through a human rights lens.[39] Yet, of the collection's eleven chapters, only one focused on health, and within that chapter, reproductive health was only mentioned once.

Reproduction is both a biological and a political project. It is biological since physical bodies reproduce. It is political since why and how people reproduce (or not) are not solely or even primarily private matters. Rather, reproduction is subject to public support *and* critique in the form of cultural images and state intervention in the form of policy and legislation. The field of reproductive and sexual health rights within the

United States remains an area of rights that the relatively recent publications on human rights in the United States have not explored adequately, even when scholars address health more generally.[40]

In the case of reproductive politics, abortion does not encapsulate the entirety of women's reproductive experiences, yet protection of legal abortion has been the most visible activity attributed to US reproductive rights organizations. Securing legislation certainly required some cultural shifts in thinking about women's bodies, which in turn was moved forward by courts. Many critics argued that the Supreme Court ruling on *Roe* was too far ahead of cultural acceptance of abortion.[41] As later cases proved, the ability to exercise the choice to have an abortion depended on the government's willingness to provide funding too. As a result, in 1976, the Hyde Amendment restricting federal funds for abortion was passed. Medicaid recipients, people incarcerated in federal prison (who are disproportionately Black and Latina), Native American women on reservations who receive healthcare through Indian Health Services, federal employees, and military personnel cannot obtain abortion through their healthcare. The Hyde Amendment, which was challenged and upheld in *Harris v. McRae* (1980), is a rider attached to the federal budget; thus Hyde is renewed each year when a new federal budget is approved. This illustrates how economics clearly underpins rights.

Various rulings have imposed further limits on who can obtain an abortion and when. For example, the 1992 Supreme Court ruling on *Planned Parenthood of Southeastern Pennsylvania v. Casey* upheld the twenty-four-hour waiting period between a woman receiving counseling on abortion and her obtaining the abortion, as well as the requirement of parental consent (or judicial bypass) for a minor seeking an abortion.[42] To secure economic rights so all people could equally choose to have an abortion would require a cultural shift from government noninterference in an individual's right to choose to have an abortion to government funding of choices, including the choice to have an abortion or to have children.

Women of color advocating around reproductive health concerns, many of whom increasingly identified as part of a "Third World Within,"[43] found themselves at odds with feminists who understood abortion rights as women's primary reproductive concern. A central focus for US women of color has been and continues to be challenging population-control ideology that marks their bodies as deviant. As the rest of this book will demonstrate, activists who came to found the reproductive justice movement were involved in the reproductive activism of the "second wave" of feminism. Yet, they voiced frustration at the continued focus on abortion to the exclusion of other reproductive issues. Abortion was certainly one of their concerns since limited access and unsafe conditions for some illegal abortions disproportionately affected poor women and women of color.[44] However, they could not separate their bodies from the context in which they were living. Thus, the social changes that these women of color sought necessarily included broader community issues that did not fit neatly into the standard reproductive activism of the era. For example, police brutality endangered Black and Latino children and was therefore an area of mobilization—and remains so.[45] Further, many of these women also saw their struggles as connected to global dynamics. A vision of liberation that was based solely on seeking change within the United States' political structure was a limited one. They wanted to look beyond resistance and survival to create conditions of thriving. A human rights approach offered one such vision.

Framing Human Rights

Social movement actors are constrained by the larger discursive context and power relations in which they make their claims. The concept of human rights exists in numerous realms, including ideals, law, and practices. The concept of human rights provides a way to frame, or talk about, the world. Frames do a lot of "work" for movements: they explain a problem (diagnostic framing), offer a solution (prognostic framing), and ideally motivate people to join the cause (motivational framing).[46] Frames condense meaning about the world, so the framing process itself is contentious as movement leaders "argue, debate, and negotiate via interactive discursive processes."[47] Thus, we cannot isolate framing activities from the larger set of discourses that already reflect power differentials that permeate society.[48] Framing is ultimately about power: who has the power to make certain claims and *be heard* in part depends on the power structure of society.

Thinking about how organizations frame problems is a useful tool with which to analyze the relationship between an SMO's membership and its interpretations of a problem, both of which are influenced by the organization's history and its members' identities.[49] There is no space in which "all things are equal" such that movement leaders can fully predict what will work for their cause at that specific time.[50] As Marc Steinberg reminds us, framing occurs in a larger set of discourses that *themselves* reflect power differentials that permeate social institutions.[51] Thus, "Unquestionably, framing is strategic, but in the focus on calculation and persuasion, frame analysts have neglected the constraints and limits that discourse itself imposes on such agency."[52] People in movements face different constraints that affect their ability and willingness to use broadly culturally resonant frames.[53] As Ferree and colleagues' research comparing the abortion debate in Germany and the United States shows, radical is relative: what is considered radical in one national context can be normative in another.[54] Indeed, dissatisfaction with the way power is distributed is a motivating source for many movement activities, which necessarily encourages radical framings by groups that want to voice their wholesale dissatisfaction with the system that produces these power distributions. These perspectives are radical *because* they challenge the current dominant discourse. So, "We should thus never expect all movement speakers to seek resonance. . . . Their radicalism lies in the challenge they pose to the institutionalized ways of thinking about an issue and the power relations embedded in these symbolic conventions."[55] What is considered radical depends on the context; thus the movement motivation for advancing radical ideas varies. For marginalized groups with less investment in maintaining or modifying the status quo, drawing attention to what they deem as a wholly unjust system may be more important than gaining entry into it. While some frames may resonate with dominant cultural discourses, seeking such resonance may go against a group's own collective identity, thereby making an otherwise "resonant" choice unlikely given its contradiction with the group's core identity. Movement leaders develop frames within a historical context, which constrains how movement actors understand a frame's relevance to their cause and ability to mobilize it in the future. Frames matter, but so does the larger discursive context from which they are drawn, the movements using the frame, and the identity of the people making claims.

In this book, I examine how the emerging reproductive justice movement moved away from preexisting frames of individual rights to reproduction, instead borrowing from international discourse to propose a reproductive justice frame linked to human rights. The US government engaged in *restrictive domestication* of human rights, whereas SisterSong engaged in *revolutionary domestication* of human rights. My theorization offers nuance to prior discussions of domestication and related concepts by clarifying the goal of the process: to restrict rights versus to expand rights. Regarding the US government's approach, my concept of domestication also differs from the idea proposed in work by some legal scholars considering human rights in the United States, such as Soohoo or sociological studies on same-sex marriage in which the authors use "domestication" to refer to the process through which countries determine how to integrate international law into their own political system.[56] I see the US government's restrictive domestication as an active process of refusal and containment, in this case around the meaning of human rights.

Through the strategy of revolutionary domestication, conversely, activists purposefully invoke supposedly global norms "back home" and push for a radical human rights movement. My concept differs from that of "vernacularization" of human rights, which anthropologist Merry introduced in her influential multisited ethnography of gender violence.[57] Levitt and Merry argue that human rights activism contains inherent contradictions: human rights discourse contains "magic" because the power comes from connection to ideas of universality that are visible in global documents, but to work its magic, the discourse needs to be articulated in ways that resonate locally.[58] They argue that international women's organizations adopt this global discourse because it offers advantages such as wider resonance and the potential to raise more funds, especially from international sources, giving the appearance of "global connectedness," which can increase international networks.[59] Their team's research on some examples of human rights work in the United States found that the social movement organizations did not explicitly refer to "human rights" or international human rights documents, opting instead to "translate" the ideas through "locally appropriate ideas and practices" such as civil rights.[60] Other researchers also find US activists uncomfortable with human rights language.[61] The case of SisterSong is different, however, because it often refused to "translate" a human rights agenda, choosing instead to leverage precisely the most radical ideas and implications of human rights discourse. They did so, furthermore, within a context in which the advantages of doing so were not clear or, I would argue, even present in the United States.

Human rights analyses often fall into two camps: theoretical debates about the origins of human rights and analysis of human rights at the policy or legal level. Case studies dot the literature, but only a handful focus on how US social movements engage with international human rights concerns. My book draws on those studies, the disciplinary diversity of which points to how little consensus there is on whose "territory" US human rights rest upon. The gap between where US sociology and its counterparts stand may seem minor, but it is important for a few reasons. First, it reflects the US exceptionalism visible in government approaches to human rights. Second, other US disciplines such as anthropology and law are decades ahead of sociology in their discussion and analysis of the many facets of human rights. Finally, in Canada and the UK, the disciplines of sociology, politics, and anthropology have covered the academic terrain of human rights extensively. US sociology remains woefully behind although that is changing. Pearce argues that sociology's foundational theorists' emphasis on the dichotomy between tradition and modernity shaped perceptions of progress, and of core debates about human rights as a solely modern concept toward which "traditional" communities must strive.[62] Conversely, Somers and Roberts posit that US social scientists' *purposeful* lack of theoretical engagement with human rights contributed to the idea that human rights were only of importance elsewhere.[63] While sociologists have conducted studies on human rights compliance (e.g., treaty ratification) and violations (e.g., genocide), they have traditionally avoided discussion of social aspects of morality and this discussion's potential to contribute to the debates about human rights. Sjoberg and colleagues suggest that sociological insights about the form and function of formal organizations, the site of extensive human rights activity (including violations) would benefit the study of human rights.[64] In particular, sociologists are uniquely qualified to illuminate the relationship between individual violators and the organizational contexts that encourage violation through implicit or explicit norms. Yet, it stands to reason that the converse is true: sociologists can contribute to the study of human rights through studying SMOs that encourage human rights protection, such as SisterSong.

I draw on several theories to explain how race and racism influence the development of movements, and offer my theory of domestication to explain a strategy for engaging human rights in the United States. My book is a theoretical and empirical contribution to the social movement literature and human rights literature precisely because I focus on *why* activists are attracted to human rights and *how* they negotiate that attraction within powerful structural and cultural barriers. Thus my work fits more with the "enterprise" approach promoted by some sociologists: "While human rights instruments frame (in practice) human rights as privileges for a generous state to grant from the top down, the human rights enterprise shifts our attention and perspective to human rights as inalienable, and subject to the will of the people rather than the state."[65] Yet, as sociolegal scholars note, the naturalization of human rights can facilitate mobilizing efforts, but legally human rights are to be struggled for and scholars should pay attention to the contours of the struggles. As US sociology enters the academic human rights debates comparatively late and begins to explore how human rights affect all aspects of social life,[66] scholars in other countries offer their own lessons learned. A Canadian scholar reflecting on the work of a US sociologist cautions against supporting the emphasis on law—"the longstanding presumption that human rights are primarily realized through law and governments"—and encourages researchers to instead pay attention to practices "to reveal how human rights norms are manifest outside the law."[67] While the legal aspect of human rights should not be downplayed, rights exist in the realm of aspiration.

One idea on which scholars appear to agree is that the idea of "human rights" exemplifies a radical approach to conceptualizing rights claims. These ideas seem quite revolutionary considering global capitalism, which intertwines nations and their inhabitants irrespective of any one individual's preferences. Human rights are about how to structure US society and relationships with each other that challenge long-held ideas about certain groups. Or, as one scholar argued,

The 1948 Universal Declaration of Human Rights (UDHR) was a complete and total breakthrough. What it achieves is an affirmation that all the others have the same rights as the people who look/talk/act just like us. (*It is easy to defend the rights of those people who look just like us, speak*

the same language, vote for the same political party, have the same kind of
work, etc.) The UDHR affirms the rights of everyone (a word that it re-
peats in every article), especially those who are different, to be accorded
equal treatment, that is, whether woman or man; regardless of age, language, citizenship; regardless of education and occupation, one has full
inalienable human rights to social, cultural, and economic rights as well
as to civil and political rights.[68]

Of course, even this quotation contains within it the underlying
assumption that produces contradiction: the phrase "those who are
different" presumes that there is a standard from which to be judged
as different. That standard is generally understood to be a White, prop-
ertied man. However, some activists acknowledge the tension between
the origins of human rights documents and the diversity of people
to whom the norms in the documents are supposed to apply. Thus,
when women of color claim human rights, even tentatively, they are
proclaiming boldly: I am just as human as the men who colonized this
country.

Methods

I first encountered SisterSong in 2006. I was a research assistant on the
Global Feminisms project, which covered a number of countries. Started
in 2002, this University of Michigan–based project focused on feminist activism in four countries—China, India, Poland, and the United
States. Partner institutions abroad coordinated video interviews of ten
feminist scholars/activists with the aim of providing the materials for
free public distribution. Each site decided on partner organizations,
interviewee selection process, and interview location. Elizabeth Cole
directed the US site, with an emphasis on interviewing activists whose
work focused on the intersection of gender and at least one other movement. Starting in 2006, I worked as a research assistant on the US site.
I helped coordinate the logistics for the last two interviews in the US
site and was provided the opportunity to interview Loretta Ross, the
national coordinator of SisterSong at the time.[69] This began a continuing relationship with SisterSong and the larger RJ movement, which has
shifted, expanded, and persisted.

The archival data on which I draw dates from the 1980s to the 2000s—over 1000 documents. The materials varied from SisterSong's internal documents such as e-mail exchanges stored on their server, to which Loretta Ross gave me full access; to their publicly distributed newspaper, *Collective Voices*; to documents from formal archives at Smith College's Sophia Smith Collection. My initial data collection occurred during the period 2007–2011 during which I conducted 58 original interviews. Starting in 2007, I conducted over two hundred hours of observation at Sister-Song events, at the SisterSong national office, and at other reproductive justice events. The first of these, the May 2007 national conference in Chicago, was both a celebration of SisterSong's tenth anniversary and an opportunity for people to see what type of work member organizations were doing. SisterSong estimates that a thousand people participated in the four-day convening. I also observed a two-part workshop that Sister-Song presented at the first US Social Forum in Atlanta in June 2007 (for which SisterSong was a member of the host committee). I attended an RJ 101 training at the Mother House (SisterSong's office), participated in SisterSong conferences, and at one point even answered phones at the Mother House on a trip to collect physical files from SisterSong's offices.

Whenever possible, I identified myself as a researcher, for example, during the group introductions at workshops. When the setting allowed, I took notes on a computer. At other times, I took notes via cell phone by text messaging myself or, as technology advanced, taking notes on the phone. Throughout the manuscript, I use quotation marks to distinguish direct quotations from paraphrasing or my analysis.

Participant observation was a critical data source that enriched my understanding of SisterSong and the broader RJ movement. Participant observation has a long history in sociological research. Whereas observation suggests a researcher who, like a lab scientist, sits physically outside the phenomenon under study, *participant* observation means that the researcher is "not merely a passive observer" and may take a role in the organization, movement, or setting under study.[70] This more active role is also what many critics (and even supporters) consider the central dilemma of this type of data collection: the ability of the researcher to affect the research site or be affected by it.[71] In the time after initial data collection, I remained in touch with many people and collected more data, which sometimes brought its own challenges (see appendix A).

There are many possible ways to tell the story of SisterSong and human rights. Even though as researchers we draw our conclusions from our data, we are ultimately producing a narrative influenced by both our disciplinary assumptions and our own social location. My training—in sociology, gender studies, and social work—and my own life experience led me to pay attention to power. Throughout the book, I attend to intersectionality, an approach to research emerging from Black feminist praxis that considers how people's experiences are constituted through multiple statuses of oppression and privilege.[72] Further, intersectionality attends to institutional structures and social processes that (re)produce inequality.[73] At points, my writing signposts intersectional analyses and yet at other times it does not, owing to the fact that the analysis is infused with intersectionality. The farther away I have moved from the initial data I collected—and shifted attention to other parts of the movement, such as helping start a reproductive justice research center in 2012—the more nuanced my understanding of these issues has become. I write with a specific set of questions that animated my initial interest, so while not everyone will agree with my interpretation, including some people present at the time about which I write, I continue to talk with people about my ideas and dialogue about what it means to engage human rights in the United States.

Structure of the Book

There are many interesting things to explore about the reproductive justice movement and SisterSong specifically. However, most are beyond the scope of this book.

Chapter 1, "Restrictive Domestication: Human Rights and US Exceptionalism," denaturalizes the nonresonance of the human rights frame in the United States by unpacking its history. I review the development of human rights in the international arena, paying particular attention to the history of efforts within the US civil rights movement to engage with the United Nations. I explain how and why the United States has since established a de facto form of US exceptionalism that largely exempts it from the very global norms it was so central in establishing. The chapter examines the consequences of this exceptionalism for human rights' general cultural resonance in the United States, and specifically for social movements therein. While the historical content of the chapter may be familiar to some readers, it is the theorization of the US government's strategy as *restrictive domestication* that provides the crucial backdrop for the rest of the book.

This chapter interweaves history and theory to explain how and why human rights constitute such a nonresonant frame within the United States, and what this has meant for social movements there. Critically unpacking this history is crucial, for it reveals how the meaning of human rights—far from being "natural" or given—has been constructed and circumscribed both in the international realm and in the United States. It elucidates, in short, the US government's strategy of *restrictive domestication*, which created the conditions under which the US reproductive justice movement and SisterSong would later operate. The discourse and practice of US exceptionalism vis-à-vis human rights has far-reaching consequences. Understanding whose interests have been served and what is at stake in these efforts to delimit the meaning of human rights sets the stage for understanding how and why it was in another group's interests to challenge that meaning. That attention to human rights developed in tandem with the United Nations is generally understood, but less well known are the ways in which their meaning was shaped from the start by the legacies of colonialism and the struggle for civil rights. I review precisely this history of contestation bound up in human rights' legal construction. Next, I focus on US exceptionalism—how it was established through a deliberate, multipronged strategy of restrictive domestication, and how the US government continues to resist efforts by various social movements to challenge it.

Chapter 2, "Pushed to Human Rights: Marginalization in the US Women's Movement," complements chapter 1 by explaining the domestic movement context out of which the reproductive justice movement and SisterSong more specifically emerged. Understanding the history of the larger US women's movement and its mainstream focus on only some reproductive rights is necessary to understand how and why SisterSong was predisposed to adopt a culturally nonresonant frame. Far from a purely rational-choice selection, SisterSong's adoption of a human rights frame was a deeply political choice that emerged from the history of marginalization of women of color within the mainstream women's movement. The chapter explores the internal movement implications of the way reproductive health was initially framed by US feminists, comparing whose realities and concerns were recognized and whose were occluded. The story is, in part, about how women of color were pushed out of the mainstream women's movement and towards both the global arena and a nonresonant cultural frame. It is, at the same time, however, the story of how women of color began to push *back*.

The first empirical (historical) chapter explains the roots/desire for something more. We see that early women of color activists had long been dissatisfied with the mainstream women's movement. That is not new, but in the space of reproductive politics, it also has a specific consequence. The emphasis on abortion by the reproductive rights movement also became the largest/most visible issue for the broader women's movement. Thus, a different approach was radical in the sense of challenging the mainstream of a movement. Of course, the radicalness is only in relation to a particular center. But the radical only looks so in relation to a center that is viewed from a particular worldview. Thus, the radicalness of one community is only deemed so from the perspective of the conservative activities of another. It was also radical to claim that the experience of women of color as women of color could inform the experiences of White women. To claim that the experiences of women who were further marginalized by race were just as valuable as the experience of women who benefited from racial privilege was also a radical act. This chapter lays out the push dynamics of the movement sector that provided conditions for SisterSong's embrace of human rights. Further, it illuminates the challenges and contestation in choosing human rights as a framing device, which have not been as visible in other accounts. This contestation is important for understanding more clearly how this movement proceeded. While reproductive movement histories make clear the external threats movements have faced, the movement's internal dynamics are just as important as, if not more important than, external pressures for understanding its nature and development over time. The dissatisfaction of women of color with the larger women's movement was the result of feeling marginalized within it, distrusting its "mainstream" organizations (whether or not women of racial/ethnic minority groups were participants), and desiring to develop analyses of reproduction that moved beyond the binaries of "pro-choice" versus "pro-life" that had become the standard discourse around abortion.

Women of color activists had participated in many movements, including the mainstream women's movement and nationalist movements. Some participated in special caucuses in mainstream organizations created for them or in women's caucuses within racial justice organizations. Some mainstream women's organizations created special posts to address the issues of women of color. Some women of color chose to develop independent organizations that sometimes included radical White antiracist feminists.[74] Still, many women of color consistently articulated that ultimately their concerns and perspectives were given lower priority.

Chapter 3, "Pulled to Human Rights: Engagement with Global Gatherings," examines key moments and dynamics immediately before and after SisterSong's founding in 1997. As chapter 2 began to highlight, SisterSong's "puzzling" selection of a human rights frame begins to make sense once we understand that women of color in the reproductive justice movement sought not simply resonance but *recognition*. The chapter narrates the formation of SisterSong, emphasizing the contingent, identity-driven nature of the process and its unfolding alongside—rather than preceding—the turn to the global arena and the discourse of human rights. I organize the chapter by focusing on international conferences at which SisterSong's founders were exposed to a new potential model for their domestic advocacy. The international arena provided such a forum and site of inspiration. Then, I discuss some of the early growing pains as activists and organizers struggled to reconcile different understandings of human rights, weighed the pros and cons of adopting them as a frame, and began tackling the practicalities of how to put the frame into action.

Chapter 4, "Training the Trainers amidst Backlash," provides a deeper examination of SisterSong's use of human rights as a discourse and framework for educating its own members. Picking up where chapter 3 left off, I draw on interviews that reveal the optimism, confusion, and tension within SisterSong and related organizations regarding the use of this framework. As discussed in the previous two chapters, there were both push and pull factors regarding the human rights approach. In this chapter I examine some of the key competing imperatives that were present in the early years of the collective, which then affected the visibility of the human rights frame. Though understandings of what human rights meant shifted and were contested over time, I highlight the emergence of a radical reaffirmation process as a more specific tactic within the broader strategy of revolutionary domestication, one that repositioned diversity within the RJ movement not as a problem but—to the contrary—as its unifying mission. Consequently, in this chapter, we see the varying ways "human rights" was embedded in these discussions. These different ideas about the origins and functions of the human rights approach impacted whether and how consistently it was used. While the approach was not always consistent in appearance or definition, it was there, which matters since these were foundational years. Further, I show how SisterSong leaders tried to work with like-minded organizations while embedded in a challenging funding climate where foundation leaders with the resources to help the organization advance human rights in the United States remained ambivalent and openly skeptical.

Chapter 5—"Marching toward Human Rights or Reproductive Justice?"—focuses on these ideas along with the realities of competing imperatives of building a sustainable women of color movement while dealing with the mainstream women's movement's continued marginalization of women of color. I do this at the movement level by analyzing the frame shift around the 2004 March for Women's Lives. The process through which movements develop their framing is contested, and the cooperation of competing organizations in a coalition can be fraught with tension. I explore how different frames were brought together, and I show that positive consequences can become a part of the social movement field even after a formal coalition ends. This contributes to the answer about the visible effects of a human rights–based coalition frame on the women's movement. This chapter suggests that even subtle deployment of a human rights frame can result in large movement gains.

In chapter 6, "Writing Rights and Responsibility," I demonstrate how SisterSong educated about human rights through various fora. As the collective shifted structure, the printed newspaper SisterSong produced and other written material were important since more people could interact with these materials at their leisure without the costs associated with travel to an event. Using examples from the SisterSong newsletter, I focus on rhetorical devices in revolutionary domestication of a human rights discourse, namely, engaging a process I term "radical reaffirmation" and leveraging the ambiguity between "social justice" and "human rights." While the focus of the chapter is on analyzing print documents, embodying the human rights framework, as happened at conferences and workshops, remained important, and as I show in a vignette, offered necessary opportunities to engage in intramovement education among SisterSong members.

In Chapter 7, "'They're All Intertwined': Developing Human Rights Consciousness," I focus on the different ways interviewees talked about their understanding of human rights or lack thereof. What emerges is a more nuanced understanding of human rights as not so much a static frame, but a continually evolving language and lens through which SisterSong participants assess movement strategies and envision future goals. After considering the role of race and space in envisioning human rights, I highlight the different metaphors members used to describe human rights as a foundation, umbrella, or thread. Then I analyze how some interviewees integrated a human rights framework into their daily practice.

Chapter 8, "'Puppies and Rainbows' or Pragmatic Politics? Organizations Engaging with Human Rights," considers how interviewees responsible for their organization's programmatic efforts talked about how these organizations utilized a human rights approach in their practice (or not). I show the complexity with which social movement organizations struggle as they balance values with the demands of the political environment. Namely, member and allied organizations had different yet overlapping audiences, who had a range of knowledge on their substantive issues (reproduction) and varying levels of receptivity, including hostility toward the human rights approach. Finally, the book's conclusion, "Making Utopias Real," shifts back out to the national level to discuss how risky human rights framing continues to be for US social movements. "Human rights" is both a catchphrase and an ideal toward which many activists claim to be working. In many respects, the human rights frame remains most important as a vision toward which movements can work, an ideal beyond easy reach, but attainable with extensive effort. This ideal provides a critical niche and a valuable toehold for leverage for some organizations, setting them apart within a highly saturated and unequal social movement sector, in which success can never be taken for granted.

1

Restrictive Domestication

Human Rights and US Exceptionalism

Human rights are a construction rather than a natural concept over which there was or is any given consensus. The scope and significance of "human rights" remains highly contested across the scholarly and activist literatures on human rights broadly and on formal human rights institutions like the United Nations specifically. Even among those relatively few scholars who consider human rights in the US context, positions vary. Historian Carol Anderson, who documents engagement by the early US civil rights movement with the United Nations, proposes that human rights are still the "prize" to be won in an approaching Third Reconstruction, which some might argue is happening in the United States now.[1] In contrast, historian Samuel Moyn identifies human rights as the "last utopia," claiming that "they have done far more to transform the terrain of idealism than they have the world itself" and thereby suggesting a less optimistic future for mobilization.[2] Questions such as where the idea of "human" began, what its defining criteria are, or what the relationship is between humans and nonhumans, while interesting, remain outside the scope of this book.[3] My focus, instead, is on how activists, mostly, and governments, secondly, grapple with the discourse of human rights.

Debate continues over when to pinpoint the origins of the concept of human rights. There is general agreement, nonetheless, regarding the history and development of the United Nations and the signing of the Universal Declaration of Human Rights (UDHR)—and, more specifically, the profound significance of the Holocaust in shaping these events.[4] Put bluntly, the Holocaust, while morally reprehensible, was not illegal at the time. There was no accountability when a government abused its people. Or, to put it another way, "massacring one's own citizens simply was not an established international legal offense."[5] After World War II, many nations debated how to ensure that the atrocities of the Holocaust could not happen again, and proposed developing the United Nations as one response.[6] In an idealized vision, the UN would serve as the institution through which governments regulated each other.

From the outset, however, determining who exactly would define human rights and how they would be enforced was a deeply contested process. Historian Grace Leslie finds that African American club women such as Mary McCloud Bethune of the National Council of Negro Women played a crucial role in pushing forward a human rights agenda. Consequently, "An interracial coalition of American women working within overlapping campaigns for peace, international understanding, racial equality, and labor and women's rights stepped forward to declare that only full human rights and an understanding of global interdependence could ensure a lasting peace. They created a vibrant women's internationalism, one determined to foster an 'international mind' among the American people and to lift the public's eyes from the national to the global stage."[7] This meant balancing competing ideologies across different movements.

At the 1945 Conference on International Organization that founded the United Nations, member states met in San Francisco to discuss the UN's foundational membership agreement, the UN Charter. The United States and Britain dominated the debates, aiming to emphasize the superiority of their democratic political system over that of communist China and the Soviet Union. China suggested adding a proposal on human rights to sections beyond the Economic and Social Council section to which it had been relegated. Secure in their control over the process, British and US representatives "decided that it was important to let the 'Chinese save face' and agreed to incorporate into the draft UN Charter three 'harmless' proposals on cultural cooperation and international law."[8] Beyond this concession, inclusion of proposals on colonialism and racial equality were resisted by US and British representatives, who worked to enshrine in the documents the structures of the global social order in which they were the dominant colonial power. Global norms and human rights were all very well, but Western powers had no interest in inviting public scrutiny of their own countries.

For the United States, discussing human rights in the global arena was tricky insofar as it drew attention to the nation's racial inequalities and internal struggles over civil rights. This fact was not lost on activists within the United States. After World War II, African Americans engaged with international human rights issues saw the UN as a space to further their claims for racial equality. When allowed, they actively engaged in the process of developing the UN. Through a combination of scholar W. E. B. Du Bois's lobbying and the US government needing good publicity around this new body, representatives of nongovernmental organizations (NGOs) such as the National Association for the Advancement of Colored People (NAACP) were added as "consultants" to the 1945 United Nations Conference on International Organization. But just as quickly as activists within the United States recognized the potential for an international discourse of human rights to be leveraged at "home," so too did US officials identify this danger and move to nullify it.

Fearful that NGO consultants and southern government officials would leave unhappy if either side received too many concessions, a high-ranking US policy advisor added what many scholars identify as the main concession that encourages exceptionalism: the domestic jurisdiction clause. Article 2(7) of the UN membership charter states, "Nothing contained in the present Charter shall authorize the United Nations to intervene in matters which are essentially within the domestic jurisdiction of any state."[9] Thus, just as another attempt at a global cooperative of nations was being developed, each national interest was being protected, undermining the purpose of a global body. The UDHR itself contains thirty articles and begins with the lofty sentiment that "recognition of the inherent dignity and of the equal and inalienable rights of all members of the human family is the foundation of freedom, justice and peace in the world."[10] It continues with veiled reference to the Holocaust and World War II: "Disregard and contempt for human rights have resulted in barbarous acts which have outraged the conscience of mankind, and the advent of a world in which human beings shall enjoy freedom of speech and belief and freedom from fear and want has been proclaimed as the highest aspiration of the common people."[11] The UDHR's preamble inclusion of freedom of speech, freedom of belief, freedom from fear, and freedom from want echoes the Four Freedoms.[12] After much negotiation among nations, the Universal Declaration of Human Rights was adopted in 1948.

These early years were critical for setting the stage for human rights policy and practice domestically and internationally. Through a compelling narrative that challenges the sanitized history of the US civil rights movement, historian Carol Anderson brings to light the abandoned struggles for human rights.[13] It is ultimately a story of the basis of the US government's restrictive domestication and the unintended consequence of the NAACP's unsuccessful attempt to leverage human rights in the initial development of the UN. The expansive human rights framework appealed to African Americans who were trying to dismantle institutionalized racism. W. E. B. Du Bois, on behalf of the NAACP, even submitted an extensive petition directly to the United Nations focusing on the hypocrisy of the US government. The petition, *An Appeal to the World: A Statement on the Denial of Human Rights to Minorities in the Case of Citizens of Negro Descent in the United States of America and an Appeal to the United Nation for Redress*, outlined the history of "negroes" in the United States, starting before slavery, and pointed to the many ways they contributed to the wealth of the nation while remaining subjugated.[14]

Unsurprisingly, the petition had little visible effect. Anderson notes that advocates wanted economic issues included in their advocacy because "it was clear to most in the NAACP leadership that without economic rights, civil liberties rested, at best, on quicksand."[15] The Cold War anticommunist climate, however, made framing social problems in terms of full human rights, including economic and social rights—rights promoted by China and Russia—too politically risky.[16] Women such as Bethune who were attuned to respectability politics risked their hard-won national standing and garnered the attention of the House Un-American Activities Committee.[17] Already-embattled African American advocates thus shifted their focus instead to civil rights—a delimited component of human rights not saddled with connotations of being "un-American." Anderson concludes, "The Cold War identified in stark, pejorative terms entire categories of rights as antithetical to basic American freedoms. It punished mercilessly those who advocated a more expansive definition and a more concrete commitment to those rights. . . . The resulting inability to articulate the struggle for Black equality as a human rights issue doomed the subsequent Civil Rights movement. . . . [T]he African American leadership was simply incapable of embracing the now-tainted human rights platform."[18] Her bleak analysis points to the risks of US movements trying to engage human rights. While Anderson's point is specific to African Americans, the larger context of the Cold War and its lasting influence applies more broadly: the juxtaposing of human rights against ideals of freedom would remain a barrier with which all movements would have to contend. Various US progressive movements have forged connections with international counterparts, from labor activists to civil rights advocates to feminist "Encuentros" in Latin America to Black Lives Matter activists' explicitly global campaign.[19] But these efforts make movements vulnerable to having their loyalty to the United States questioned. The history of "human rights" in the United States constrained how post–civil rights movements could engage with the discourse for framing and organizing purposes. That these stories have largely been unknown and unexplored by scholars until the past decade or so highlights the difficulty in excavating alternative discourses.

In the decades following the UN's founding, countries continued to debate how precisely to institutionalize the ideals contained in the UDHR. Various attempts were made to draft international treaties, with limited success. Instead, in 1966, after almost two decades of discussion and revision, two separate covenants were adopted.[20] The International Covenant on Civil and Political Rights (ICCPR) focused on rights such as voting (i.e., "first-generation rights"). The International Covenant on Economic, Social, and Cultural Rights (ICECSR) focused on rights such as education (e.g., "second-generation rights"). The language of "generations" produces confusion by suggesting that one set of rights was achieved, then another set envisioned, when, practically speaking, they are interrelated.[21] While both the covenants were completed in 1966, they were not adopted until 1976. Together, the UDHR and the covenants are sometimes referred to as the International Bill of Human Rights. The extensive time taken to draft the documents, combined with the ten-year lag until formal adoption, hints at the intense conflicts left unresolved by these documents. From the beginning, some government officials and representatives of nongovernmental organizations wanted the UN to succeed whereas others wanted the UN to fail. Because both supporters *and* opponents of human rights contributed to drafting key documents, legal scholar Christopher Roberts notes that the documents themselves are "social texts" that reveal power differentials among nations, requiring us to read them with an eye toward the continual conflict over the meaning of rights.[22]

Establishing US Exceptionalism

The domestic jurisdiction clause was of importance in the United States, as it laid the groundwork for continued US exceptionalism and restrictive domestication. Not surprisingly, many have argued that US leaders unduly influenced the shaping of early human rights documents. The debate about the development and applicability of universal standards has raged for decades.[23] However, the structure of the UN is such that many nations were involved in developing the initial standards—and continue to debate them. Thus, the perception that there is a single standard decided by a single nation and applied to the rest is only partially correct. Governments can make proposals, and even if the majority accepts a proposal, governments, including those that supported the passage of the proposal, can attach their reservations. The domestic jurisdiction clause makes it possible for any recognized nation to turn away from its own social problems and focus instead on criticizing other nations. Thus, exceptionalism is embedded in the UDHR for all nations.

Exceptionalism operates in three key ways. Canadian historian turned politician Michal Ignatieff identifies three types of exceptionalism in which present-day governments engage: the government (1) signs treaties, then exempts itself (exceptionalism); (2) is biased when reviewing its own behavior and that of its allies in comparison to others (double standards); and (3) does not recognize international human rights law in its own courts (legal isolationism). To be clear, many governments engage in some or all these practices. Yet, as Ignatieff points out about the United States, "No other democratic state engages in all three of these practices to the same extent, and none combines these practices with claims to global leadership in the field of human rights."[24] The United States thus holds the dubious honor of "winning" in all categories of exceptionalism. Meanwhile, US presidents have claimed leadership around human rights, irrespective of their party affiliation. To put it another way, the US government consistently operates hypocritically, irrespective of the leader in office.

President Jimmy Carter, arguably the US president whom people most clearly identify as formalizing the United States' relationship to enforcing human rights, stated in his 1977 inaugural address that "because we are free, we can never be indifferent to the fate of freedom elsewhere. Our moral sense dictates a clear-cut preference for those societies which share with us an abiding respect for individual human rights." Carter's idea of human rights rested on the assumption that the United States as a nation was "free" and that people in foreign countries needed their human rights protected. A few months later, Secretary of State Vance began a speech about human rights by noting, "Many here today have long been advocates of *human rights* within our own society. And throughout our nation that struggle for *civil rights* continues."[25] Here, in a speech delineating the administration's approach to human rights, Vance both recognized *and* conflated human rights and civil rights, with the latter being identified as the domestic equivalent of the former. This is vexing, as these areas of rights are related but cannot substitute for each other. Vance said the administration's three-part definition of human rights included "the right to the fulfillment of such vital needs as food, shelter, health care and education," which "can be violated by a government's action or inaction—for example, through corrupt official processes which divert resources to an elite at the expense of the needy, or through indifference to the plight of the poor."[26] This suggests an interest in economic rights. Nevertheless, the United States itself was not fulfilling "vital needs" as Carter's administration claimed other nations needed to do. Years later, when Carter accepted the Martin Luther King Jr. Nonviolent Peace Prize, he reiterated his view connecting the United States' morality with foreign policy: "This administration is working to restore America's moral authority in the world. As I've said before, human rights is the soul of our country's foreign policy. And as long as I'm President, America will continue to lead the struggle for human rights."[27] Carter's comments implied that human rights were not part of the "soul" of US *domestic* policy, yet the United States was to lead other nations. This is an example of restrictive domestication, as it placed the focus of US human rights activities on social problems *outside* the United States.

Other presidents continued to engage in restrictive domestication. As political scientist Mertus shows, US policymakers equate human rights primarily with US values and practices, rather than with the broader view of human rights as understood internationally. Mertus likens the US government to a used car salesman using a "bait and switch" technique in which the US government's claims for a desire to advance human rights are used to "sell" the public on various controversial acts such as unilateral military intervention abroad.[28] Thus, when US policymakers talk about human rights, they often do so with a "vision of human rights [that] accommodates double standards" in which the United States does not have to meet the same standards it insists upon for other countries.[29] This leads to the US government articulating a hypocritical rhetoric, championing civil and political rights for its citizens, while generally ignoring other rights (e.g., economic and social) domestically, and criticizing other nations for their failures to protect human rights.[30] Restrictive domestication offers a tempting view of human rights: that individuals can achieve human rights through exercising an individual right to vote or that a legal guarantee of equality under the law is the most important way to access human rights. People can live under equally horrible conditions while still retaining their civil rights. Thus, a focus on civil rights does not require human flourishing. Further, restrictive domestication does not address what people need in order to exercise these rights on a practical level. It does not, for example, address how reliance on market logics has eroded the right to *have* rights, even for formal citizens.[31] As more sociologists turn their attention to human rights as relevant to the United States, their insights offer us more ways to consider the nuances of human rights. For example, Berkovitch and Gordon consider that according to a traditional measure of political rights, the right to vote, the United States appears to have a high standing. But when they analyze the legislation that disenfranchises (former) felons who are disproportionately African Americans, the picture differs.[32]

US schools provide another example of how the government engages in restrictive domestication. US schools do not offer standardized mechanisms of educating students about the UDHR and human rights such as the right to food. Any education around human rights that happens is in scattered doses that result from individual teachers' motivation to expand their repertoire, but is not woven into the core fabric of education.[33] This is in contrast to rituals such as the Pledge of Allegiance that children recite every morning, from primary school through high school, equaling thousands of schools across the country saying words that reinforce commitment to the United States and God.[34] Without standard ways to learn about human rights, people in the United States lack opportunities to develop the consciousness that would allow them to imagine an entitlement to rights that shifts their thinking and might mobilize them to action and advocacy.

The US government's focus on first-generation human rights (i.e., civil and political rights) has influenced its specific states' focus on human rights, again forcing framing these rights in limited ways. When "human rights" is used in the United States, it is often as a synonym for civil rights protected by US law. For example, in the period under study, twenty-two US states had state agencies with "human rights" in their title (e.g., New York State Division of Human Rights). These agencies focused on discrimination in public arenas (such as employment and housing) based on statuses protected in the Civil Rights Act of 1964. These protected statuses include race and sex, although some states did address sexuality or single-parent status.[35] Thus, even though these agencies addressed civil rights violations—a subset of the range of human rights violations understood as such in *international* discourse—they largely restrict "human rights" to "civil rights."

As of this writing, the US government has a Bureau of Democracy, Human Rights, and Labor, the website for which plainly notes, "Promoting freedom and democracy and protecting human rights around the world are central to U.S. foreign policy."[36] Democracy is identified first and "democracy" is repeated in some form three times in the successive brief description. Further, the bureau is under the jurisdiction of the undersecretary for civilian security, democracy, and human rights, which focuses on issues of "security," the language used for military and counterterrorism operations. Hence this position "leads State Department efforts to prevent and counter threats to civilian security, such as violent extremism, mass atrocities, and weak governance and the rule of law. The seven bureaus and offices reporting to the Under Secretary advance the security of the American people by assisting countries around the world to build more democratic, secure, stable, and just societies."[37] The undersecretary oversees other agencies, including the Bureau of Counterterrorism and Countering Violent Extremism and the Office of Global Criminal Justice (focused on "mass atrocities"). According to these examples, as far as the US government has been concerned, human rights is a matter of *foreign* policy, with the US government having the responsibility of promoting human rights outside the United States by ensuring a specific form of governance, namely, democratic. In the period under study in this book, some of these offices had different names and functions. However, overall, the US government has promoted a vision of human rights that focuses on exporting its vision of democracy, increasingly connecting the vision to antiterrorism efforts that require military force—all while shaping human rights discourse to meet the government's needs.

A common conclusion in the past decade's flurry of scholarship on human rights in the United States is that the US government and policy elites promote "first-generation" civil and political human rights such as voting, while largely ignoring "second-generation" economic and social rights such as the right to adequate work.[38] This makes the United States a hostile environment for US social movements explicitly attempting to advance a range of human rights. Consequently, the United States is an acutely confounding example. We should remain cautious about idealizing other governments and their approaches to human rights. But ultimately the United States is the context in which US social movements primarily engage. Ultimately, the US government's splitting the "generations" of rights provides the basis for exploring the unusualness of domestic human rights activism.

Some suggest that the tension between civil rights and more expansive human rights results from the fact that the initial goal of civil rights legislation was, primarily, to protect African Americans and women from active discrimination rather than passive neglect. The important difference between civil rights and human rights is that civil rights do not go as far as human rights because civil rights "are merely adjustments to a systemic structure that is otherwise entirely acceptable," whereas "human rights" suggest the necessity of a supportive social structure even if that means systemic change.[39] However, this downplays how radical civil rights were to many, as evidenced by the intense violence faced by civil rights–era activists. Further, the continued backlash against codification of basic civil rights shows how radical that subset of human rights remains a century after African Americans began mobilizing around those issues. Still, paying attention to the panoply of human rights allows us to consider the difference between *reforms* to a government's operations and *systemic* changes to the underlying logic of the government's operations. The former offers a liberal approach to social change while the latter is a revolutionary approach.

Contemporary Restrictive Domestication

The US government's historically ambivalent relationship to human rights has continued to the present. Some researchers find that Americans support a version of human rights—but only in *other* countries.[40] According to an Opportunity Agenda report on human rights in the United States, a 1997 poll found that only 8 percent of Americans could name the UDHR. At first glance, the Opportunity Agenda's 2007 report a decade later offers a hopeful view of possibilities for future human rights organizing in the United States. The explicit goal of their study was to assess people's readiness for framing issues in terms of human rights. The study claims, "Human rights as a concept is clear and positive for Americans" and "the public places many social justice issues in a human rights framework."[41] However, the report's last two conclusions offer a less optimistic view, stating, "Perceptions of the role of government complicate human rights communications" and "communicating about international treaties is a long-term challenge."[42]

The Opportunity Agenda study also found that people had low levels of awareness of international treaties. The authors observed that some respondents "*were pleasantly surprised to hear that such mechanisms exist*, while others expressed concern that such laws had not produced many benefits over the years. Still others worried about the effectiveness of international bodies, or the wisdom of applying a single standard to all nations."[43] Opportunity Agenda's study identified two sets of people: people unaware of international mechanisms but hopeful about them and people aware of international mechanisms and skeptical.

Perhaps it is easier for an untested idea to seem more appealing than the tested idea that has been proven imperfect. Opportunity Agenda suggests that the public is comfortable with the term "human right" because respondents believed in basic rights as demonstrated by high agreement on certain phrases. Yet, as with many ideals, while the theory is appealing, actual practice remains contested: "Americans are generally receptive to a discussion of human rights violations in the U.S. but are divided on some specific applications."[44] The tension between theory and practice makes engaging human rights an uphill battle for US SMOs. The Opportunity Agenda report and other studies reach to some of the deeper problems with organizing around human rights in the United States: people are simultaneously unclear and skeptical about the international components of such rights.[45] Yet, one of the key reasons the UN was developed was to provide a mechanism for international connection. Activists outside the United States who are engaged in human rights activism shift these dynamics when they rely on these elements to demand government accountability within a world system of political relationships.

Human rights discourse contains many contradictions, providing both a powerful tool to reinforce ideas of US superiority and also offering "almost limitless possibilities for imagining alternatives."[46] Policymakers and activists use human rights discourse to further their respective goals, which can often be at odds. As more groups claim human rights, the boundaries of "human rights" are expanded, which means that on a practical level so are the potential categories of people protected under them.[47] This may seem obvious to some readers, but politically, the idea is radical and presents a challenge to the US system—arguably, in particular. The US government has restricted human rights domestically, in part through tainting them as dangerously foreign. Understood thusly, human rights become both a weapon and a shield; accusations of violations are lobbed against other nations, even used to justify military interventions, while the notion of human rights is used as a shield staunchly oriented outward, deflecting attention from human rights abuses within the United States, such as labor exploitation or removal of voting rights. Thus, activists advocating for deep change in the form of revolutionary domestication must contend with the ways that restrictive domestication has been and remains the dominant discursive structure that underlies the social movement sector.

US Social Movements and the Human Rights Frame

World polity theorists argue that human rights have gone from a set of proposals supported by a select group of countries to a set of norms, institutions, and laws with which governments must engage to some degree in order to appear legitimate. This is the case because human rights are contained in a "model" that experiences "a considerable amount of consensus" globally.[48] Nation-states are *expected* to support human rights to demonstrate their legitimate membership in the club of "good" states that promote democracy; how they interpret rights and whether they meet this expectation are different and significantly more complicated questions.[49]

Human rights discourse remains powerful for non-US activists because it represents a system supported by the internationally recognized UN; it also produces expectations within countries and provides a means for people and movements to challenge the impunity of the state.[50] The gap between nation-states' statements supporting human rights and states' practices provides space for SMOs to demand that nations live up to what may have been initial "empty" promises, resulting in many successful social movements to affect and improve social conditions.[51]

In international contexts, social movements engage with human rights by relying on the "boomerang effect," which describes the way domestic social movements appeal to international bodies to exert pressure on their governments and gain concessions in their own country.[52] Underlying this theory is the assumption that the relationship between national and international political arenas can create opportunities where they did not previously exist, particularly in the realm of human rights. However, the ability to create pressure is limited when the offending government (the United States) is one of the most powerful and has structurally positioned itself beyond those pressures. The US government's outsized role in UN interactions is a problem not just for grassroots advocates but also for high-level officials. After his term as UN secretary-general, Boutros Boutros-Ghali wrote a book—*Unvanquished:*

A United Nations–United States Saga—the title of which illustrates the difficulty of negotiating the politics of the UN and the United States.[53]

We can see the US government's dualistic relationship with the discourse of human rights and the way it engages them. Some of its inward-facing activities include wielding power as a permanent member of the UN Security Council and dismissing the human rights of its citizens. Some of its outward-facing activities include claiming protection of human rights as justification for military intervention or criticizing the human rights record of other countries. For example, under President George W. Bush, justifications given for pursing the Taliban included its treatment of women. The US Department of State's Bureau of Democracy, Human Rights, and Labor released a report a month after the September 11, 2001, attacks on the World Trade Center. Human rights and a supposed concern for women emerged: "With one of the world's worst human rights records, the Taliban has perpetrated egregious acts of violence against women, including rape, abduction, and forced marriage."[54] While the violence was indeed a problem, claiming that women in other countries needed the United States' rescuing exemplifies a "bait and switch" that ignored how war would unequally affect these women. The US government has traditionally not been concerned with international pressure since its moral standing globally has little effect on its ability to operate economically or politically. These are just a few of the historical reasons why the United States is an exceptional case if activists were to focus on the "boomerang" style of advocacy.

Many progressive social movements continue to seek inspiration for visions of the world they want to create. This was particularly important in the reproductive justice movement, where founders had a long history of fighting against the world they did not want. Attending to movement actors' multiple identities and experiences helps us understand varying ways movements can successfully operate at what Crenshaw termed the "political intersections," where many people reside.

2

Pushed to Human Rights

Marginalization in the US Women's Movement

In examinations of the US women's movement, scholars note that an emphasis on "waves of feminism" (e.g., first, second, and third) privileges visible activism by White feminists in explicit women's organizations, leaving out the many other people who engaged in politics in varying forms.[1] Common historiographies of the US women's movement note that popular texts such as Betty Friedan's 1963 *The Feminine Mystique* drew attention to the sense of entrapment that domesticity and motherhood engendered for racially and socioeconomically privileged White women who embodied the educated housewife experiencing "a problem that has no name" (later identified as, among other things, emptiness and lack of purpose).[2] White women argued that due to gender oppression, they did not have choices: they were to marry and have children. Feminists such as Friedan did speak to concerns that a sector of US women faced and directed those concerns to creating organizations such as the National Organization for Women (NOW). However, as other authors demonstrate, the assumption that the experience and desires of White, heterosexual, middle-class wives could express the experience and desires of all women was short-sighted at best.

Contraception remained illegal for married couples until the 1965 *Griswold v. Connecticut* ruling that established a right to privacy. The right to privacy would be the basis for the argument for federal legalization of abortion in the 1973 *Roe v. Wade* ruling. Since the *Roe* ruling, mainstream pro-choice organizations have remained in lockstep battle with the pro-life movement. As Luker details, the *Roe* ruling led to an almost overnight shift in consciousness for many pro-life advocates, who quickly committed themselves to developing a cohesive countermovement to repeal any gains made by the "abortion rights" movement.[3] The *Roe v. Wade* ruling was in part the result of decades of activism by "uneasy allies" of feminist activists and medical professionals.[4] Mainstream reproductive rights organizations' partnerships to improve their strategic position and legislative success undermined long-term possibilities for building coalitions that could engender broader cultural change. For example, NOW and the National Women's Health Network's alliance with Zero Population Growth (ZPG) on abortion issues put them at odds with racial justice advocates who decried environmental organizations' rhetoric, which they viewed as continuing the eugenic thinking of earlier decades. ZPG and similar organizations supported abortion access on the argument that overpopulation caused resource depletion. Further, these organizations encouraged the use of permanent birth control to curb the birth rates of "hyperfertile" communities in the United States and the "Third World."[5] These types of alliances were reminiscent of earlier coalitions forged by birth control advocates, such as Margaret Sanger, who sought support from wealthy eugenicists.[6]

Differing approaches to issues such as forcible sterilization offer one example of the splits in the women's movement about what constituted a valid issue around which to focus organizational and movement attention. Sterilization was a controversial issue that sometimes placed women on different sides of the debate. Record keeping on state-sponsored sterilization varied, but some statistics suggest that in the early part of the twentieth century, upwards of 150,000 people (majority women) were forcibly sterilized with the support of the federal government as late as the 1970s.[7] In the 1970s, some particularly egregious cases of forced sterilization made national headlines. One was that of the twelve- and fourteen-year-old Relf sisters. Medical personnel administered birth control to the sisters. The two girls were eventually sterilized with the "consent" of their illiterate mother, who was told that her daughters were receiving additional birth control.[8] The *Relf v. Weinberger* ruling came months after the *Roe* decision legalized abortion. The responses to the details of this case, and to forced sterilization in general, have varied among women along lines of race and class, demonstrating the complexity of the underlying implications of these procedures and the concerns of population-control ideology that led some seemingly liberal activists to support abortion and sterilization.

A specific example of this tension is visible in the 1976 Western Regional Conference on Abortion, cosponsored by doctors and numerous organizations, including the National Abortion Federation and ZPG. The conference had enough resources to include a banquet dinner featuring Sarah Weddington, the lawyer who successfully argued the landmark *Roe v. Wade* case. Of all the scheduled talks, only one featured a speaker to provide an "ethnic perspective" on abortion.[9] The speaker, Jessica Luna, offered her comments as a self-described Chicana feminist addressing what she saw as key problems with abortion rights activism. She noted that Latinos and Blacks were diverse, just like "you"—White people of the audience who performed abortions. She spoke of a "triple jeopardy" of race, gender, and class discrimination. It is not that minority women were not concerned about abortion being legalized. Minority women were disproportionately poor, and poor women disproportionately bore the consequences of the illegal abortions that were performed by unqualified personnel.[10] To ensure cultural relevance, she encouraged employing more Chicanas in abortion clinics. Further, she noted that as a mother of six children, five of whom were sons, she felt "terror" at some feminists' characterization of all men as "monsters" and implored the audience to include Chicanos at "every level of decision-making in the abortion movement."[11] Luna being the lone speaker designated to speak about "ethnic" issues is not surprising when one looks at other conferences at the time, but underscores the White dominance of the field of reproductive activism and legal advocacy.

Activism around abortion and sterilization continued along parallel lines, only sometimes intertwining, although practically, women of different races continued to have differing reproductive experiences. The Hyde Amendment of 1976 demonstrated how economic resources were a critical part of the ability to exercise certain codified rights such as abortion. Representative Henry Hyde, who proposed the amendment, was unabashed in his desire to eradicate legal abortion: "I certainly would like to prevent, if I could legally, anybody having an abortion: a rich woman, a middle-class woman or a poor woman. Unfortunately, the only vehicle available is the Medicaid bill."[12] The amendment restricted federal funding for abortion except in cases of life endangerment, rape, or incest. States could use their own funds for Medicaid recipients to obtain an abortion in other cases, but this further left the most economically vulnerable people to the whims of their state.[13] The 1977 death of a young Latina student, Rosie Jiménez, became the first case around which radical feminists rallied to point to the way Hyde disproportionately affected poor women. Jiménez, who used Medicaid, had to decide between paying her college tuition or obtaining a legal abortion. She chose tuition, opting for an illegal abortion, after which she developed an infection and died within a week. English and Spanish posters produced by the Reproductive Rights National Network for a "pro-choice vigil" included a picture of Jiménez and the exhortation to ensure that proposed changes to state funding for abortion were prevented because "we must work to keep abortion a right for all, not a privilege for some." That remains an elusive goal.

Historically, working together, women of color and poor White women fought for access to a range of reproductive healthcare. Around sterilization, they advocated for explicit informed consent procedures. They wanted mandatory waiting periods because of the mounting evidence that women who opted for sterilization had been coerced through financial inducements that required sterilization for them to obtain welfare benefits. Or, as in the case of the Relf sisters or women whose doctors sterilized them immediately after childbirth, women had the decision made for them.[14] Middle-class White women, on the other hand, found that when they requested to be sterilized, paternalistic doctors doubted their decision and would often make the process more difficult, leading activists from those communities to demand loosening restrictions for sterilization.[15]

Women of color and their allies continued to seek satisfactory ways to address the complexity of the factors that affected reproductive experiences. A letter from the newly founded Committee for Abortion Rights and Against Sterilization Abuse (CARASA) to Eleanor Smeal, president of NOW, reveals that the differing perspectives on sterilization generated public debate among "sisters."[16] CARASA acknowledged that increased regulation of sterilization could curtail individual women's reproductive rights. CARASA and many women of color argued that increased regulation would, nevertheless, protect economically disadvantaged women in the United States.

The letter differentiated between the theoretical opposition and the practical implications of government noninterference around some reproductive options: "Sterilization abuse . . . occurs because population control advocates, individual doctors, social welfare agencies, teaching hospitals and others believe that they have the right to determine which women will limit the number of children which they will have and the method by which this will occur. Far from being patronizing to a particular group of women, strong sterilization guidelines protect the rights of all women against these anti-choice forces. This means that a woman's choice to be sterilized is made with full information and with no coercion."[17] While sterilization had the same medical consequence for these diverse groups of women—termination of the possibility of future childbearing—the challenges faced by women of different statuses vary due to complex racial and class stereotypes that impact public health policy.

Economic status continued to impact women differently. The *Harris v. McRae* Supreme Court ruling in 1980 upheld the Hyde Amendment. The majority opinion offered that "whether the freedom of a woman to choose to terminate her pregnancy for health reasons lies at the core or the periphery of the due process liberty recognized in *Wade, it simply does not follow that a woman's freedom of choice carries with it a constitutional entitlement to the financial resources to avail herself of the full range of protected choices.*"[18] Further, the majority opinion reaffirmed, "Although government may not place obstacles in the path of a woman's exercise of her freedom of choice, it need not remove those not of its own creation, and indigency falls within the latter category."[19] Translation: the government did not create the problem of poverty, which led to Medicaid use; therefore, the government was not required to resolve Medicaid's lack of abortion coverage. The government was not required to take an affirmative stance to help economically vulnerable people.

Three justices, including Marshall, wrote a dissent arguing that Hyde was essentially punishing poor women. The dissent opined that Hyde was "a transparent attempt by the Legislative Branch to impose the political majority's judgment of the morally acceptable and socially desirable preference on a sensitive and intimate decision that the Constitution entrusts to the individual. Worse yet, the Hyde Amendment does not foist that majoritarian viewpoint with equal measure upon everyone in our Nation, rich and poor alike; rather, it *imposes that viewpoint only upon that segment of our society which, because of its position of political powerlessness, is least able to defend its privacy rights from the encroachments of state-mandated morality.*"[20] Power and politics were intertwined for women differently; thus the Hyde Amendment would affect women differently.

The data bears this out. Besides people who use Medicaid, people who use federal healthcare in some form are subject to the Hyde

Amendment's restriction: federal employees and their dependents, military personnel and their dependents, Peace Corps volunteers, Native Americans using Indian Health Services, low-income residents of Washington, DC, federal prisoners, and disabled people who rely on Medicare are a few of the examples. The Hyde Amendment is renewed each year.[21] Hyde was—and many advocates argue continues to be—a clear example of the limits of legal approaches. A rich woman using private insurance and a poor woman using federal government insurance both have a legal right to an abortion, but only the first one can be assured she can obtain the abortion.[22] Rights remain symbolic if, practically, people cannot exercise rights. Senator Hyde was explicit in his wish to ban all abortions, but he was not legally allowed to do so. So, he used legislation to exercise part of his wish on a vulnerable group: poor people. Thus, many women of color deduced, a culture in which the government did not take responsibility for its citizens' health and well-being equally was a limited context in which to advocate. As law was not separate from society, to get more effective laws required a more supportive culture. How could they expect to shift US culture if the women's movement still focused on the experiences of a relative few?

Invitation to Be Silent: Engaging the Mainstream Women's Movement

Event fliers and organization newspapers from the late 1970s/early 1980s further illustrate the different approaches to reproductive politics by mainstream organizations and organizations that considered themselves radical challengers to this mainstream. Organizations like the National Organization for Women challenged normative cultural expectations of domesticity by insisting that women should only become mothers "by choice." The membership brochure of one NOW chapter included a drawing of a woman holding a smiling baby surrounded with the words "Motherhood By Choice . . . Not By Chance. NOW is the time when *you* can make the difference."[23] The delights of motherhood were clear even as the organization emphasized "choice."

Conversely, organizations like CARASA suggested that women of color were having the choice to become mothers taken away from them due to forced sterilization. One CARASA flier advertising a talk began with a statistic: "25% of Native American Women Have Been Sterilized." The flier went on to note that the speakers would be "speaking on forced sterilization and radiation effects on reproductive health, followed by a discussion of U.S. genocidal policies toward Native Americans and other people of color."[24] The flier specifically linked reproduction and environmental hazards ("radiation effects"), while invoking a shared history of government mistreatment toward communities of color. CARASA's event was held in conjunction with the national Long Walk for Survival to bring awareness to Native Americans' disadvantaged status in the United States. The reference to genocide on CARASA's flier highlights how, for these women, forced sterilization was not just an issue of the disruption of an individual woman's ability to reproduce; rather, forced sterilization was a larger issue that put a whole community's future survival in jeopardy.

For these activists outside the mainstream, addressing individual women's reproductive experiences required understanding reproduction in the context of inequalities of class and race that produce significant variation in whose reproduction was/is controlled through such measures. Thus, reproduction was framed as a community concern, not just a concern of autonomous women. In reflecting on a 1986 Philadelphia conference, Between Ourselves: A Reproductive Rights Forum among Women of Color, a member of the Organization of Pan Asian American Women wrote about her doubts about taking her children to the event. She was pleasantly surprised that "the broad range of sponsors of the conference which included religious and international organizations, was somewhat reassuring as well as intriguing. It didn't appear to be a propaganda conference by women's libbers." That convening included discussion of abortion and forced sterilization, and the author noted, "The fact white women dominate the issue [of reproductive rights] does not render it a non-legitimate issue."[25] These are but a few of the examples of women of color and poorer women advocating for a more nuanced analysis of reproductive health.

Women in mainstream organizations who were specifically tasked with addressing diversity lacked support. In 1987, Loretta Ross organized the first Women of Color and Reproductive Rights conference when she was working as director of Women of Color Programs at NOW. Characteristically, Ross brought her own perspectives to the position: "And we actually shifted the paradigm, because Ellie [Smeal] thought my job was to bring Women of Color into NOW. I thought my job was to figure out why women of color hated NOW. . . . So [laughs], it was . . . I became more like an ombudsman than a recruiter, which I thought was a really important distinction."[26] Such a distinction was useful in designing programs that resonated with women of color.

The conference, advertised as "for and about women of color," would provide the first national forum in which women of color could discuss their feelings of marginalization from the pro-choice movement, share experiences of working on sometimes-controversial reproductive issues, and strategize for the future.[27] Some of the advertised workshops focused on racism in the pro-choice movement, Medicaid funding for poor women, and genetic technology. The NOW letter sent to event cosponsors noted how women of color in the reproductive rights movement had been marginalized, so one of the conference aims was "to place the concerns of women of color in the forefront of the pro-choice debate."[28] This was a laudable goal.

Yet, documents provide evidence that despite NOW's promotion of the inaugural conference, infrastructure issues persisted. Internal memos from three months before the conference include Ross's request for interns because she was "quite desperate for some assistance on this conference," as she was "swamped with hundreds of details." Additionally, she had "no idea" of the budget within which she had to work.[29] Ross noted that one potential intern, a woman of color, decided not to intern due to the costs incurred by an unpaid internship.[30] Further, Ross suggested that NOW chapters should more aggressively publicize the conference and provide scholarships for women of color to pay the twenty-five-dollar conference fee.[31] That three months before a *national* event, the sponsoring organization had not worked out key "details" like the budget suggests disorganization at best and apathy at worst.

Still, attendance surpassed expectations, with four hundred attendees converging on Howard University, a historically Black college that had donated the space. Over thirty workshops were presented. Shirley Chisholm, an outspoken Black feminist, former presidential candidate, and one of NOW's founders, served as a plenary speaker and made a surprise appearance at another part of the conference. Notes from the 1987 NOW conference indicate that other groups were included that had not traditionally been included in mainstream "choice" conversations.

NATIONAL ORGANIZATION FOR WOMEN

WOMEN OF COLOR
AND
REPRODUCTIVE RIGHTS

MAY 15-17, 1987
HOWARD UNIVERSITY
WASHINGTON, D.C.

Topics Include:
Medicaid Funding for Poor Women
Teen Pregnancy
Religion and Reproductive Rights
Abortion and the Genocide Question
Racism in the Pro-Choice Movement
Women of Color Working for the Right Wing
Speaking with Young People about Sex
Medical Abuses Against Women of Color
Family Planning vs. Population Control
Male Responsibility
Genetic Screening and New Technologies

NATIONAL CONFERENCE FOR AND ABOUT WOMEN OF COLOR

REGISTRATION: $25 (sliding scale registration and child care available)
Site accessible to the physically challenged

FOR MORE INFORMATION CONTACT :
Loretta Ross (202) 347-2279
National Organization for Women
1401 New York Avenue, N.W., Suite 800
Washington D.C. 20005

EVERYONE IS WELCOME TO PARTICIPATE IN THIS EXCITING CONFERENCE

PLEASE SEND ME MORE INFORMATION ON THIS CONFERENCE !!

NAME _____

ADDRESS_____
CITY/STATE/ZIP_____

ORGANIZATION_____

PHONE (DAY)_____ (NIGHT)_____
            area code   area code

Figure 2.1. Flier for Women of Color and Reproductive Rights Conference (1987)

For example, a small group of pro-life African American women pick-eted outside the conference. The women were invited in and conference notes include some of the items discussed, such as whether abortion was racist. Even though conference attendees were generally in support of reproductive rights, their willingness to engage in dialogue with the "opposition" suggests that they were unwilling to stay on one side of the "pro-choice debate." Even though conversations about reproduction often pointed to a male-dominated society as the problem, conference notes also show that men attended. One conference assessment noted that there was "lots of praise for the inclusion of men working on repro-ductive rights."[32] This event appeared to be a success by various mea-sures. However, the full extent of NOW's resources does not appear to have been made available to support the conference, highlighting the disconnect between a mainstream organization's stated desire to wel-come women of color and its practices.

Even after publicly supporting such a landmark event and creating special positions for women of color such as the one Ross filled, NOW was met with skepticism. In early July 1988, Ross wrote to organizations that were part of a women of color coalition around Title X (federal fam-ily planning funding) to suggest a retreat to discuss the issues women of color faced organizing around reproductive rights and to discuss de-veloping a network. A few weeks later, Sharon Parker, the chair of the National Women of Color Institute, responded to the request:

> I received your July 7 memo to members of the Title X coalition and, after reading and re-reading it, am quite disturbed. . . . [A]lthough I think that you intended to facilitate the progress of the Coalition with your memo, to me it signals strife. And with *my* experience with NOW, I see real and perceived co-optation of a true women of color issue by the organization. Let me explain why: (1) simply sending your memo on NOW stationery implies more officiality than you probably intended; (2) the content of the memo implies that no women of color reproductive rights project exists . . . and (3) given past experiences such as the Women of Color and Reproductive Rights conference last year (earlier this year??), I see little support for the RCAR [Religious Coalition for Abortion Rights, now Re-ligious Coalition for Reproductive Choice] and lots of visible organizing [by] your NOW office in this arena.[33]

Parker objected to perceived duplicating efforts and working with mainstream organizations. Parker suggested that NOW could be organizing around the issues, but she remained concerned that the women of color coalition would be "co-opted" by a national organization.[34] Further, Parker suggested that some issues were "true" women of color issues. Explicit in Parker's letter is the articulation that NOW was not a women of color organization. NOW may have had women of color involved in its founding (such as Chisholm) and in membership, but this did not mean it could effectively advocate for women of color—at least not from Parker's perspective. Here, we see evidence of a continuing tension that emerges throughout this book concerning the organizing efforts of women of color: wanting the support of mainstream women's SMOs, yet simultaneously distrusting their motives.

The liberal approach to abortion protection that focused on an individual woman's right to privacy was critiqued even during the second wave of feminism. Even though abortion was a primary issue that invigorated some feminists of these decades, criticisms of this emphasis emerged from minority women, whose reproduction was historically viewed as negative. Further, White allies offered critical analyses on the limitations of a movement focused on protecting the "choice" to access abortion. One long-time reproductive activist-scholar, Marlene Gerber Fried, observed, "In trying to hold on to past gains, the pro-choice movement has failed to pursue new ones, either by solidifying its own membership or speaking out to the public. *Roe v. Wade* was not the first step of a feminist agenda for reproductive control; it turned out to be the *only* step, defended by appeals to the right to privacy—the importance of keeping the government out of our personal lives—and to religious tolerance."[35] Thus, this "step" ended up being taken repeatedly, thereby producing well-worn path dependence.

After the 1989 *Webster v. Reproductive Health Services* decision, the National Right to Life Committee began a concerted campaign to restrict abortion through enacting legislation limiting access in particular situations.[36] In response, reproductive rights groups narrowed their focus to maintenance of *Roe v. Wade*, while battling for territory against the pro-life movement, which continued to gain an increasing share of the "hearts and minds" of the US public, according to polls and media reports.[37] In a few decades, abortion went from being an issue not addressed on presidential platforms to being a divisive moral issue that determined how various constituents voted.[38] Consequently, with abortion remaining one of the most contentious issues in contemporary politics, many other reproductive concerns remain peripheral to the mainstream reproductive movement agenda—a situation increasingly critiqued by women of color.

Journalist Saletan outlines how the major abortion rights organizations such as the National Abortion Rights Action League (NARAL), NOW, and Planned Parenthood moved toward pro-choice conservatism to appeal to voters who supported abortion rights for libertarian reasons—noninterference by government. This approach relied on downplaying a radical feminist argument for abortion. As Saletan writes, "So instead of talking about women's rights, the activists portrayed abortion restrictions as an encroachment by big government on tradition, family, property. When the issue was framed that way, many voters with conservative sympathies turned against the anti-abortion movement, and the balance of power turned in favor of abortion rights. From the beginning, the alliance was unstable."[39] When observing results from Arkansas focus groups in 1986, pro-choice leaders also recognized that latent racism and classism affected people's responses to questions around abortion. In Saletan's account, Lynn Paltrow, then an attorney at the American Civil Liberties Union (ACLU) of New York and therefore holding some power, remained the lone voice arguing against the pro-choice activists taking a conservative route. Further, she continued to argue in favor of fighting for public funding of abortion. Mainstream pro-choice groups, however, took a different tack, continuing to emphasize abortion as individual choice, devoid of context, in which a woman and her doctor would decide what was relevant.[40]

Evidence of domestic discontent that pushed radical activists toward human rights can be found in SisterSong founders' reflections on experiences with other mainstream organizations. In an interview, SisterSong founder Luz Martinez recalled her tumultuous experience with NARAL. She described her initial enthusiasm about becoming a board member:

> A White woman that was a strong factor as an ally wanted to nominate me to the NARAL board, and I didn't know NARAL, I didn't know the organization. But she said, "There are very few women of color." I think there were a couple and she wanted to try and change that. So, I said, "Sure.

Let's try to do something." Because I also was interested in mainstream diversifying and broadening their agenda and I'll do the work I can. So, [I was] thinking I could make a change, and this woman who worked in communications, [an] African American woman. . . . She is great, and she had actually arranged the training for women of color working in reproductive health, media training. It was excellent. I told her about getting on the board and this is what I'm going to do and it's going to happen. It felt like she was patting me on the head—OK, you can go try that—because she knew NARAL. She had worked with NARAL before.[41]

Martinez's description of her involvement with NARAL begins with the encouragement of a White ally. She was excited about possibilities for increasing the diversity of the organization. She faced what could be perceived as a patronizing attitude from another woman of color skeptical about the possible results of Martinez's efforts.

Martinez then described the difficulty she and allies faced when they would bring the concerns of women of color into NARAL's planning:

So for months, years, the time that I was there, I would keep pushing. My first meeting, I thought the [African American] pediatrician would be there. I met with her. She was going to support me, but for family reasons, she wasn't at this first meeting that I was at. And I looked around the room and something came up and I thought, "Oh, shit, she's not here and I guess I have to bring it up." They were talking about some media thing that they were working on, or some research they were doing, and I didn't see where they were including women of color. So I had to speak up. So I talked about that, the importance of it, and having women of color interviewed as well, and bringing all the different issues in. I know they didn't pay attention to me but I said it. But that was the beginning. And there were other White women on that board that were also wanting to make some changes. So everybody speaking out, everybody speaking up. And I remember the meeting where the board finally made the change. Not the commitment but the change . . . but we were all there, three or four women of color, and all these White women. There might have been a couple of men, too. But the issue came up. We need to do something about diversifying the board. We need to put something in the bylaws about this. Oh my god, that discussion was crazy. People were crying and screaming and the board chair said, "If you do that, that will be the worst thing that can happen to NARAL." Wow.[42]

According to a later e-mail exchange, one of NARAL's funders suggested the proposal about the board composition.[43] Martinez's time with NARAL "pushing" the leadership suggests her own personal commitment to reproductive rights. Yet, her experience also highlights issues women of color consistently faced when working with mainstream organizations—issues that my interviewees said they continued to face and that I hear at events in the present day. First, there was the issue of visibility—if women of color were not in the room or were there but chose not to speak, then an issue was not addressed. Second, leaders of the mainstream organization were inconsistent when it came to taking actions that could shift the long-term structural operations of their organizations. Nevertheless, even though various women of color voices were not heard, there was a collective effort that included some White and male allies interested in changing the way the mainstream organizations operated.

Of course, while not all leaders in mainstream organizations articulated fears that diversifying their boards would be the "worst thing" to happen to their organization, the existence of these comments indicates that increasing the racial diversity of organizations was not an easy task. NARAL was not the only mainstream organization that women of color criticized.

In many of my interviews, concerns about marginalization in other organizations were raised. "Sonya," a Latina interviewee, worked for a Planned Parenthood affiliate during the 1990s. During that time, she also created an informal group for Latina women to discuss sexual health. In our interview, she recalled the difference between how she felt among that group of Latinas and how she felt about the mainstream "family planning" movement:

> *It didn't really resonate with me because there was a whole cultural piece and spiritual piece that was missing for me.* And so when I, when I was around the table with all of these [Latina] women . . . it wasn't missing. It was there. . . . [T]here was no hit and miss there. And there were no questions asked. We just, we were a collection of women who were determined and compassionate and didn't have to make assumptions. *And so that's what I was really thinking about [when I said], "We have our own voice." And let*

us stand for who we are. Please don't open the door and ask us not to come in, so to speak, you know what I mean? (Sonya, Latina, emphasis added)

Sonya continued to speak about the importance of "culture" and how she had tried to integrate culturally specific ideas into the Planned Parenthood programs by drawing on her own experience. In Sonya's recollection, when she became pregnant as a teenager, she only encountered the assumption that her pregnancy was a "deficit" from people outside her Latino community. Sonya felt that young Latinas she counseled would resist health education that reinforced dominant stigmatizing discourse about teen pregnancy.[44] Sonya's earlier comment was echoed in several data sources: many women of color felt they were invited into mainstream spaces to add visible racial diversity, but when they wanted to voice concerns over their different reproductive experiences, their perspectives were literally silenced or not taken seriously. Yet, as Sonya described, in settings that women of color created for themselves, many felt they could finally bring up how identities other than gender influenced reproductive health, without worrying that their ideas would be dismissed. In these spaces, the "door" was physically *and* conceptually "open" to women of color.

An article in the Black Women's Health Initiative's (BWHI) newspaper pointed to continuing difficulties with the National Organization for Women.[45] The BWHI's frustrations over attempts to talk with NOW's leaders about the representation of women of color in an upcoming national march were explained. That the BWHI felt ignored was obvious: "Somehow, the national N.O.W. leadership failed to understand, even after three face to face meetings, beginning the first week of December 1992, the need to seriously consider and address the concerns and criteria we presented regarding our participation in the march. *Quite simply, we demanded they move beyond rhetoric, start practicing what they preach concerning inclusion of women of color.*"[46] The BWHI emphasized a gap between the claim of a mainstream organization to want to diversify racially, and the organization's practices, which kept that diversification from becoming a reality. While there were many examples of women of different racial backgrounds working within mainstream organizations, integrating diverse perspectives in mainstream organizations remained a persistent problem. Women of color organized in support of access to abortion, yet many wanted to broaden understandings of reproduction. As discussed in the introduction, the reproduction of particular groups of women (and men) has systematically been discouraged, as demonstrated through the historic state-supported practice of forced sterilization for women of color and the more recent criminalization of birth by drug users.[47] Yet, the mainstream reproductive rights movement largely failed to take up issues surrounding a right *to* parent.

Even though many examples of historical misunderstandings and frustrations between women of color and White women exist, some White women have served as crucial allies in creating the opening for a new analysis to bring together different movements. Marlene Fried of Hampshire College's Civil Liberties and Public Policy Program discussed details of Ross's "consultation" with the program that would include attending an April conference, writing a letter for the newspaper, and helping to arrange internship for Hampshire students. Fried wrote,

> We are interested in connecting with students at southern colleges and are interested in connecting with students of color. Certainly use your judgment in finding students to attend the conference. The criteria of commitment to reproductive rights and anti-racist work makes sense. . . . One more thought: Betsy [Hartmann] and I have been talking with Judy Norsigian and Norma Swenson [cofounders of the Boston Women's Health Collective, which published *Our Bodies, Our Selves*] about a collaborative project between us on women/feminism, environmentalism and population control. In a nutshell it seems that some environmental groups are putting out that overpopulation is the cause of environmental destruction—their solution population control. We would like to: talk with feminists; research environmental groups to find out more about what they are saying, thinking, doing in this area; bring feminists together to deal politically with these groups.[48]

The excerpt highlights how some White feminists did prioritize developing connections between seemingly disparate social movements. In this case, the connections proposed were between the reproductive and antiracist movements (ostensibly at the behest of Ross) as well as the reproductive movement and the environmental movement (per Fried).

The focus on challenging population control discourse remained important since the discourse continued to circulate. Eventually some explicit population control organizations closed. Others changed their names, such as ZPG, which is now Population Connection,[49] giving support to the assertion by critical geographer Jenna Loyd that after some public opposition, "The family planning–population control hegemony emerged relatively unscathed."[50] Mainstream women's organizations could generally not be trusted to offer critical views of the assumption in various liberal circles: overpopulation was a problem that could be solved through controlling women's reproduction. This would be a continuing tension during that era of feminism and persists into the present.

Women of color working in the area of reproductive politics continued to attempt to develop regional and national networks of solidarity. For example, the Southeast Women's Health Network aimed "to get more Southern women involved in *national and international activities* that affect women's health."[51] The network members included individuals and both women of color and general women's organizations: Sister-Love Women and AIDS Project (a founding organization of SisterSong), the National Black Women's Health Project (a "foremother" of Sister-Song), the National Women's Health Network, the Feminist Women's Health Center, the YWCA, and the National Organization for Women.

An example of a previous national network was the Women of Color Coalition for Reproductive Health Rights (WCCRHR). The coalition included groups such as the National Asian Women's Health Organization, the National Black Women's Health Project,[52] the Latina Roundtable on Health and Reproductive Rights (which became the grant agent for the initial SisterSong project), and Women of All Red Nations, an established Native American women's organization. One document noted that the multiracial coalition aimed to "design and implement a common agenda that influences policy, research, and education for reproductive health rights issues *as broadly defined by women of color, for women of color, from our perspective and on our terms.*"[53] The WCCRHR influenced both the reproductive health and rights activism of women of color and women of color in other movements engaging in human rights activism.

In sum, there were many examples of the persistent challenges women of color faced working in and with mainstream women's organizations. These challenges partially emboldened their initial interest in creating different organizations and a new movement that could advance an expanded understanding of reproductive politics. Specifically, an expanded analysis would more fully reflect the experiences of women whose lower socioeconomic status and racial marginalization resulted in a reduced ability to make the same choices afforded to other women.

In contrast, alternative organizations focused on a range of reproductive needs that are dependent on structural supports that human rights emphasize. "Choice" became the dominant way to talk about women's reproductive possibilities because it "evoked women shoppers selecting among options in the marketplace—[and] would be an easier sell; it offered 'rights lite,' a package less threatening or disturbing than unadulterated rights."[54] As neoliberal logics began to dominate policymaking, the emphasis on "choice" fit with the way Americans felt and continue to feel is the ideal way for government to interact with its citizens: with limited government interference (i.e., negative freedom). However, "interference" held different implications for different groups of women and, therefore, some proposed solutions around reproductive health benefit some women more than others.[55]

Consequently, one of the most pressing questions contemporary reproductive justice activists foreground is the myriad ways in which "noninterference" encourages some women's childbearing, while discouraging others'. Few scholars address the ways women of racial minority backgrounds and poor women have historically faced disproportionately negative consequences resulting from attempts to control reproduction. As a result, activism by women of color around reproduction-related issues may not look like the efforts by women who face discrimination based on only one oppressed status. In practice, the organizing of women of color is likely to address multiple aspects of their identities simultaneously. Thus, their efforts might include campaigns around racial justice (e.g., activism around rising rates of incarceration) or environmental issues (e.g., protesting toxic dumping in poorer communities, which creates an unhealthy neighborhood for children), instead of focusing exclusively on traditional reproductive activism. Women of color and their allies continued to seek satisfactory ways to address the complexity of the factors that affect reproductive choices. Some felt that engaging human rights discourse would encompass that complexity. International spaces, however, would also prove to have their own complicated dynamics of representation.

3

Pulled to Human Rights

Engagement with Global Gatherings

Women of color who were dissatisfied with the limits of domestic reproductive rights activism were also seeking other forums in which to advance their perspectives. Sociologist Sylvanna Falcón provides a rich account of how women of color continued to engage with the United Nations, working within its structures to address global racism and its effects in combination with patriarchy.[1] Some of the international events at which SisterSong founders exchanged ideas were United Nations conferences—such as the Conference on Women in Nairobi (1985), the Conference on Population and Development in Cairo (1994), and the Fourth World Conference on Women in Beijing (1995).

In preparation for the 1985 Conference on Women in Nairobi, a number of meetings were held to familiarize potential participants with the process of UN meetings. These meetings included women like SisterSong founder NKenge Touré, who became involved with the Black Panther Party at a young age, activism that "cost her a high school diploma."[2] After marrying a party member, changing her name to Nkenge, and having a child, Touré focused on advocating for women's role in Black nationalist politics. Upon moving to DC, Touré was involved in many projects and worked at the DC Rape Crisis Center for over a decade alongside Ross. Showing a commitment to Pan-African politics, Touré and Ross organized the International Council of African Women, which focused on engaging US Black women with the Nairobi meeting.

Challenges Nairobi attendees faced included travel logistics whereas other challenges emerged about how women with opposing political views, such as Israeli and Palestinian women, could come together.[3] Influential Black women's healthcare advocate Byllye Avery, who founded the Black Women's Health Initiative (Project), assembled a group including Charon Asetoyer,[4] Luz Martinez,[5] and Nkenge Touré, all of whom would be involved with SisterSong's founding and early development meetings. Nkenge identified Nairobi as her most formative learning experience up to that point, which is quite telling considering her range of political experiences before that meeting. In an interview, I probed Touré about why Nairobi felt so formative:

> Before I went to the conference, I mean, certainly, you know, I was aware that there was something called human rights . . . I hadn't really looked at it or thought about it in terms of how to really integrate it into my work, or how to make a connection between . . . between human rights and, say, violence against women. . . . [S]o it was a process that made me, you know, begin to think much more about that and be much more aware . . . [S]ome of the things that have been proposed by the United Nations that certain countries like the United States were not taking up and . . . not embracing on behalf of its citizens, and particularly its female citizens.[6]

Nkenge also reflected on how seeing the scope of organizing that women were engaged in internationally offered inspiration: "I mean, it just was another kind of an affirmation to the work that we were doing, that women all over the world were struggling to empower ourselves to have our human rights recognized, to end gender violence and that basically so many of the things that we . . . we're looking at in the United States, women were looking at in other places . . . that they were . . . we thought more developed [in their activism] than women in the United States."[7] Thus, over a decade before founding SisterSong, some leaders had exposure to international human rights advocacy. It is important to note that even with their prior involvement in radical politics in the United States, they still had much to learn around human rights. Consequently, when Touré later served on SisterSong's Management Circle she brought this perspective with her.

Early Efforts at Making Women Human

In the mid-1990s, US feminists focused on the idea of "women's rights as human rights." Many feminist authors challenged the private/public distinction. Feminist human rights activists insisted that gaining access to the public sphere while leaving the public/private distinction untouched would disadvantage women who were predominantly relegated to the private, or domestic, sphere.[8] Feminists argued that government's constructing women's experiences of abuse as "private" issues allowed governments to separate these problems from "real" human rights violations, even when they resulted from explicit state action (e.g., political imprisonment). It was particularly difficult for feminist advocates to separate categories of human rights since they merged in real life: "The patriarchal narrative which divorces the economic and social framework from the political and civil framework generates a story of 'civility' and citizenship that neglects the socioeconomic structures in which women's subordination occurs."[9] They argued, for example, that son preference, employment discrimination, family abuse, and other gendered violations occurred with the state's tacit permission. The tendency to tolerate these violations as manifestations of "culture," feminists argued, absolved states of their responsibility to stop these acts. Bunch argued, "Sex discrimination kills women daily. When combined with race, class, and other forms of oppression, these daily harms constitute a deadly denial of women's right to life and liberty on a large scale throughout the world."[10] These scholars questioned whether women were even "human," as people perpetrated human rights violations against women without consequence.[11] Feminist scholars argued that addressing "second order" rights such as economic rights remained especially important for women because they formed a "part of a larger socio-economic web that entraps women, making them vulnerable to abuses which cannot be delineated as exclusively political or solely caused by states."[12] Thus, attention to upholding "first-order" rights such as voting, while important, should not come at the expense of upholding other types of human rights, such as socioeconomic rights.

The realities of socioeconomic constraints and opportunities are a critical, often hard to change, element of women's lived experiences, reproductive and otherwise. As one scholar noted, "While the acquisition of rights is by no means the only solution for the worldwide domination of women by men, it is an important tactic in the international arena."[13] The existence of human rights discourse does not solve all inequality because a number of mechanisms combine to produce systematic injustice. However, this quotation highlights the expansive potential of human rights, particularly in considering the aforementioned positive rights, which contain government obligation to provide resources for people to access these rights.

Some scholars suggested that strengthening corrective legislation would be the path down which women's human rights activists would turn.[14] For example, around the issue of violence against women, women's groups throughout the world had mainstreamed efforts to combat women's experiences of violence. Campaigns such as 16 Days of Activism Against Gender Violence, started in 1991, represent a win for many women's advocacy groups since human rights documents and laws that men developed only addressed violence by the state in the public realm. After a concerted effort by activists globally, the UN formally recognized the issue of violence against women and has continued to support advocacy efforts and evaluations around this issue. Around sex trafficking, different feminist ideologies led to different approaches to activism, sometimes leading to unlikely coalition partners.[15] Ultimately, the creation of the Trafficking Victims Protection Act, which was developed on the assumption that sex work was inherently exploitative trafficking, deepened conflicts between transnational women's groups ostensibly all working toward women's equality. Yet, there was *some* type of action by many nations and internationally around what was being deemed a social problem worthy of attention.

Reproductive health stands in stark contrast as a "women's issue" that has not been accorded sustained activism or support from the United Nations. Reproduction is an important area of inquiry when one is analyzing human rights debates because "the physical territory of this political struggle over what constitutes women's human rights is women's bodies."[16] Despite major development entities such as the World Bank recognizing that promoting reproductive health improves a country's outcomes on a range of measures (e.g., education), the UN eschewed specific inclusion of reproductive health in the Millennium Development Goals.[17] Whereas at the UN level there is a yearly campaign that focuses on stopping violence against women and a UN Declaration on the Elimination of Violence Against Women, an equivalent does not exist for reproductive issues. The UN does have goals relating to reducing maternal mortality.[18] Still, there are not yet advocacy groups successfully advocating for setting aside special weeks to acknowledge the number of women who have died in childbirth. Contraception and abortion remain controversial at the UN level—information about them is buried in UN documents.[19]

The link between sexuality and morality motivated many societies to limit women's reproductive options, making reproduction an increasingly common, yet controversial site of state intervention.[20] Turner proposes that debates over women's human rights emerged due to changing economic conditions in which (some) women gained more economic and social power.[21] While changing social contracts afforded more people freedom in choosing partners without family or state input, these freedoms led to heated contests around rights.[22] As people's anxiety about their vulnerability increases, social groups attempt to control private aspects of other people's lives. This lack of headway is not surprising when we consider that "women's reproductive health raises sensitive issues in many legal traditions because it relates to human sexuality and affects the moral order. . . . This traditional morality is reflected in laws that attempt to control women's behavior by limiting, conditioning, or denying women's access to reproductive health services."[23] Further, unlike rights such as voting, reproductive rights, including abortion rights, are not rights previously held by men and then extended to a different group.[24] So, advocacy claims cannot be argued from a place of equivalence with men.

Even in supposedly "advanced" nations like the United States, access to reproductive health services remains limited. For example, President Obama's 2009 efforts to include women's health as central to healthcare reform faced resistance for various reasons—including claims of declining morality and the costs of coverage. Even if reproductive health had a larger presence in international human rights documents and law, it is unclear what impact this would have on US domestic policy as the US government has had a strained if not adversarial relationship to some types of human rights, such as "second-order" socioeconomic rights, as discussed previously. With each nation-state having its own agenda for promoting specific human rights, onlookers would expect that the promotion of a range of human rights would probably come from the public sphere, through the sustained efforts of nongovernmental organizations.

Recent research suggests that coalitions between grassroots activists and legal experts can provide activists with tools to leverage human rights.[25] Yet, a limit of those efforts is that legal and technical expertise offered by elites continues to take precedence, while justice is relegated to being a goal of grassroots activists. Further, there is some evidence that staff of human rights organizations have moved away from their prior focus on creating a widespread human rights culture in favor of working with a select group of other elites.[26] Despite these challenges, there is evidence that a human rights frame is gaining in popularity in the United States because this analysis encourages marginalized people to work collectively to challenge inequality under the rubric of gaining wider human rights that go beyond the limited rights supported by any particular government.[27]

On one hand, it is surprising that SisterSong chose human rights to frame and provide a linkage. On the other hand, this choice is not surprising when we consider its constituents' general social marginalization, and consequent skepticism about the social order. While the US government had an integral role in the history of developing the official meaning of human rights through document crafting, in the contemporary moment, the human rights perspective offers a radical framing in the US context for many historical reasons.

Some SisterSong founders did have more experience with United Nations procedures. Asetoyer noted the relationship Indigenous groups have with the United Nations, which goes back to the UN's founding. Indigenous nations had formal structures that facilitated maintaining that relationship:

> You know, there were indigenous people that were at the formation of the UN, and the original charter for the UN, and so, there's always been an indigenous presence there. I spoke at the UN back in the '80s, the early '80s, pre-Nairobi, and a lot of indigenous women before [then also spoke]. We've been lugging our bags to Geneva and to New York for many, many years, with the formation of the Working Group on Indigenous Populations and through that forum, and through the World Health Organization and that forum as well, doing international work, and with tribes to the south and tribes to the north. So, working on the national level is probably the newest area for us in the mainstream. But we've been working nationally and internationally amongst ourselves, meaning other indigenous organizations and tribes and so forth with other women's groups and stuff, for a long, long time.[28]

Asetoyer's remarks show different levels of familiarity with UN processes. Asetoyer describes continued engagement with Indigenous issues at the international level broadly and the UN specifically (Geneva and New York), and with other Indigenous people nationally, including other women's groups. Here is an example of how some SisterSong founders had direct and continuing experience with formal human rights institutions like the UN. This type of experience could make human rights feel more tangible to some founders than to others who had not been to these spaces.

Naming "Reproductive Justice"

The newspaper produced by the Black Women's Health Initiative, *Vital Signs*, featured an article that pointed to an interest in the global aspects of health. In "Reproductive Health Is a Global Concern," the author pronounced, "Reproductive freedom is a fundamental human right that not only includes the freedom to have or not have children but the right to have the means that would enable women to make these choices."[29] This phrasing foreshadowed SisterSong's language around reproductive justice. The initiative would continue to influence SisterSong in scope and language.

How exactly did the phrase "reproductive justice" come to be? The "herstory," told at the events I attended and in published documents, is that twelve Black women gathered in a hotel room.[30] As Ross describes it, the term was developed to describe "reproductive health integrated into social justice"[31]—or, as she and some others have said, "reproductive rights married to social justice."[32] In the United States, there is little language with which to talk about activism around reproduction outside of the "pro-choice"/"pro-life" dichotomy. Activists' frustrations with this false dichotomy are partially responsible for the development of the reproductive justice movement. "Reproductive justice" offered a more accurate description of the novelty of the emerging movement's explicit grounding in an argument for a broader concept of reproductive justice, not just reproductive choice, which continues to be associated with abortion access.[33] Two of the women in the hotel room later held leadership positions in SisterSong—Toni Bond (Leonard) and Loretta Ross—highlighting the link between the nascent reproductive justice movement and what would become SisterSong.

Cairo Sets the Stage

In reflecting on preparatory meetings before Cairo, Black Women's Health Project activists criticized US policymakers for paying attention to international population policy while ignoring domestic population concerns. Investing in funding international health interventions, albeit oftentimes with eugenic assumptions, while disregarding minority health access, was ironic. More specifically, activists argued that the United States' "donor posture" resulted in focusing on efforts in donor countries to the elision of discussion of US women of color, particularly African American women.[34] In a statement that was ostensibly focused on the Cairo conference, activists drew on the history of US civil rights activism: "Had the African American struggle been based on human rights principles, the war on poverty of the 60s would've had development at its base."[35] Of course, as discussed in the introduction and in chapter 1, that was not possible for various geopolitical reasons out of the control of early activists. Yet, Forte's allusion to history points to some activists' awareness of how previous generations of activists—and policy—shaped their movement environment.

The draft Platform for Action released in May 1994 included limited use of the word "abortion," and even that was controversial. Further, the platform connected resources and population: "Around the world many of the basic resources on which future generations will depend for their survival and well-being are being depleted and environmental pollution is intensifying, driven by the unprecedented growth in human numbers, widespread and persistent poverty, social and economic inequality, and wasteful consumption. New ecological problems, such as global climate change, largely driven by unsustainable patterns of production and consumption, are adding to the threats to a future."[36] While many reasons were given for resource depletion, the first was the "unprecedented growth in human numbers." As part of the preamble, these concerns are foregrounded in the report. Another section of the platform connects these ideas, as demonstrated in its title: "Interrelationships between Population, Sustained Economic Growth, and Sustainable Development."

Gender equality was only explicitly addressed starting in section 3. Reproductive issues were embedded later in the report in section 7, where a tenuous link between rights and health was made in the section title: "Reproductive Rights [Sexual and Reproductive Health] and Family Planning." Whereas there was a clear "interrelationship" between population and development, the brackets around "sexual and reproductive health" suggest that achieving those forms of health were only *maybe* necessary for achievement of reproductive rights and appropriate family planning.

After the 1970s, population control organizations had ostensibly fallen out of mainstream US favor. Thus, the 1994 UN International Conference on Population and Development in Cairo served as a reminder to some activists that government officials still supported the idea that controlling women's fertility—rather than eliminating structural inequalities—could solve a host of social problems ranging from malnutrition to war.[37]

While US women of color had many stories of marginalization and exclusion from the mainstream women's movement, they also articulated the feeling that, at times, they also experienced exclusion when they attempted to engage in international women's organizing. The Ford Foundation, which would later provide crucial start-up funding for the SisterSong collective, sponsored a delegation to attend the Cairo Conference on Population and Development.[38] Luz Martinez, a Sister-Song founder, reflected on her Cairo experience. She recalled that when delegates reviewed the initial documents circulating in preparation for the meeting, they realized that the documents did not mention women of color in the United States. Martinez suggested that that exclusion prompted the women of color delegation to develop its own proposals:

> And I remember asking a White woman that did international work and saying, "Well, what about women of color in the US?" And she said, "Oh, no, no. This is about women in developing countries." And I couldn't understand why. . . . We took it [their document] to all of the delegates, especially the American delegates, and we had excellent support from some of the delegates, the American delegates. . . . So, what we said to them—because everybody else was taking care of abortion, all kinds of stuff was going on—we said to them, "We want the inclusion of 'women of color in developed countries.'" They took that on, even a couple of White women that supported us and what we were doing, so they took it and pushed it through and we got it. . . . Simple. Simple. But that was historical.[39]

Martinez's narrative suggests that these delegates found themselves in a familiar situation: in a setting that was supposedly open to all women, specific groups of women had already been excluded from the conversation. With "everybody else taking care of abortion," many other issues were not being addressed. This story points to a paradoxical situation experienced by women of color in the United States: the draft documents for the UN assumed human rights violations occurring outside "developed" nations. Yet, since the late 1960s, women of color in the United States had argued that they comprised a "Third World Within." Despite being in the "First World," their social status produced experiences and health outcomes like those of people living in "undeveloped" nations in the "Third World."[40] Far from being "simple," the inclusion of US women of color in these documents required extensive negotiation. They fought because inclusion was symbolically important for them as it acknowledged their unique status in the United States, while also making the documents relevant for future organizing with women of color in the United States.

Charon Asetoyer remembered that during the Cairo meeting, Native American women joined with other women to confront "mainstream" US women's organizations for their continued emphasis on abortion, which was creating a negotiation "bottleneck."[41] The bottleneck meant that other reproductive issues were neglected as the mainstream women's organizations continued to object to the positions of the US government and the Catholic Church (represented as the Holy See) on abortion. Asetoyer recalled, "They were challenging the Holy See, but keeping that conference bottlenecked with that one issue. There's a lot more issues than abortion. When you're looking at population issues globally, abortion is not the only issue. That's what I meant: broaden the agenda, look beyond that one mainstream issue."[42] Broadening the agenda interested women from other countries as well. For example, Black women in Brazil were organizing around reproductive health, identifying concerns about the government-sponsored sterilization programs. For those women, Cairo's population conference was also important, as was an analysis that linked the public and private domain. They wrote that "the state has basically come to treat reproduction as a public issue, and the means of sustaining life—housing, health, education, food and work—as a private matter. Understanding this role reversal is crucial at this juncture in preparation for the World Population and Development Conference III. . . . *Reproductive freedom is essential for those ethnicities that are discriminated against.* Therefore, we must fight so that reproductive decisions are made in the private realm, with the state guaranteeing reproductive rights and ensuring healthy conditions for sustaining life."[43] They wanted the state to guarantee the conditions that would make a range of reproductive choices possible, including legal rights, while ensuring that individuals got to make the choices, not the government.

As globalization expanded and technology increased possibilities for interaction across borders, women's groups worked with each other. For women's groups outside the United States, there is evidence that they coalesced into a larger movement that "became increasingly intertwined with carriers of global culture such as the UN."[44] For US groups, however, restrictive domestication continued to pose a challenge to organizing efforts. Cairo was important for many activists who identify the changed discourse around reproduction that emerged from the meetings as critical to future advocacy efforts. However, as others have noted, the "Cairo consensus" is not settled. In a reproductive technology roundtable, scholar and activist Andy Smith challenged the idea of Cairo representing a major shift in policy: "I would dispute the assumption that Cairo shifted the discourse from population to reproductive health. At Cairo the population paradigm remained. It was simply described in more benevolent language. The impact of Cairo was that people know to use different language, but the assumption that the cause of the world's problems is poor people's ability to reproduce has not fundamentally changed. Dangerous contraceptives are still promoted in third world communities and communities of color in the United States."[45] Ethnographic research like Jade Sasser's excavates how population control advocates shifted to using "empowerment" language to mobilize a new generation of young activists who surveil their own reproduction and that of other people, under that logic that their individual efforts will mitigate climate change.[46] Contemporary population control logic ignores upstream factors that affect the environment, such as corporations that pollute the air or the consumption patterns of the global North, which largely rely on production of material goods from the global South. These experiences have been constructed internally as part of the organization's development. For example, in the minutes of a 2002 Management Circle retreat, under the "History of SisterSong" heading, there is a note: "Luz Alvarez Martinez told story about Ford [Foundation] funding for ICPD and the omission of the needs of women of color in the U.S. from the discourse."[47] Still, symbolically, Cairo is an important event in the history of the emerging reproductive justice movement's turn toward human rights as exemplified through SisterSong's efforts.

Of the twenty-three participants in the official women of color delegation to the Cairo conference, four would later participate in the early organizational meetings of SisterSong, while others would become involved in other reproductive health and rights projects.[48] For example, the newly created Women of African Descent for Reproductive Justice (WADRJ) coalition wrote President Clinton in support of his surgeon general nominee, Dr. Henry Foster, an obstetrician/gynecologist.[49] They identified themselves as the same group that had advertised in the *Washington Post* the year prior to support inclusion of comprehensive reproductive healthcare in Clinton's efforts at healthcare reform. While there was overlap between WADRJ and the group that coordinated the advertisement, Women of African Descent on Health Care Reform Coalition, names matter. WADRJ noted their concern for the ob/gyn's nomination for two reasons. First, antichoice Republicans were already opposing him due to his having performed abortions. WADRJ argued for a different interpretation of his abortion provision and its relationship to teen pregnancy: through his "combatting the problem of adolescent pregnancy with creative, compassionate, common sense approaches," Foster had "deterred abortions not encouraged them."[50] Second, they claimed that when Clinton's African American nominees faced opposition, his administration failed to offer them continued support.[51] Thus their concerns were about both the content of the nominee's activities and political support for him.

Twenty-one individuals and organizations signed the letter. One of the signatories, Toni Bond, would go on to start African American Women Evolving, one of SisterSong's founding organizations.[52] Another signatory, Loretta Ross, would go on to work with the new National Center for Human Rights Education and then become SisterSong's first national coordinator, a position she held for over a decade. To say that Ross believed in the cause of human rights would be an understatement. She encouraged many US activists to engage with global convenings, including taking some of them to Beijing.

Long-time activists in multiple movements have discussed the importance of the 1995 Beijing conference in their understanding of human rights as a relevant issue for their organizing. The Stanley Foundation sponsored a preparatory meeting in April 1995, Bringing Beijing Back: Designing an Implementation Strategy. A letter from a foundation representative makes clear the challenge of US activists treating the Beijing conference as an opportunity in the same way that women's activists outside the United States considered it.[53] Based on the letter, it appears that the meeting participants did not meet the formal goal of outlining a common approach to leveraging the Beijing conference to advance rights in the United States. Rather, some of the discussion at the meeting had focused on the merits of Beijing as a location. Accusations of hypocrisy emerged since an international human rights meeting was to be held in a country that was a well-known violator of human rights. However, with the location selected months prior and the Beijing date nearing, these seemed to be, in retrospect, futile discussions. Yet April meeting attendees apparently agreed that after Beijing, "No matter what the degree of government commitments to implementation, resources will be limited, demanding new and creative partnerships with sources of private financing; . . . the inclusivity of organizing in the international forum is questionable and greater attention to more effective linkages between the grass roots and national and international NGOs is required[;] and . . . the lessons learned and strategies shared through the international process need to be more effectively disseminated to women organizing in their local communities, while local strategies need to be more effectively amplified at the transnational level."[54] They could identify the barriers. They were trying to think ahead about what Beijing could offer in the struggle to mitigate the hostile political environment.[55]

In one article that featured interviews of women of color who attended the Beijing conference, the women "described the sense of global solidarity, pride, and affirmation that they experienced in Beijing. This sense of affirmation had greater resonance, because of the sense of siege that pervades the political environment in the United States."[56] This affirmation was also critical to recognizing the implications of the United

States' role in the oppression of women from other countries. Beijing played a pivotal role in the understanding of many US feminists of color regarding how marginalized groups could effectively integrate human rights into their work to challenge the fundamental organization of society.

Beijing served as another key site for raising US women's consciousness of how global power dynamics affected reproductive futures. Due to the efforts of women of color at Cairo, the official Beijing documents referred to "women of color."[57] In preparation for Beijing, the US Women of Color Delegation to the UN Fourth World Conference on Women (USWOCD) produced its own document, *The U.S. Women of Color Statement on the Status of Women*. The delegation explained its interest in the UN conferences:

> The USWOCD is dedicated to educating the public about the legislative and governmental mistreatment of the poor, and to giving voice to women and underrepresented communities of color. Without such input, the gender and racial bias will continue in domestic policies and will continue to extend into U.S. international policies of population, development, and human rights, which most affect the so-called "Third World," whose population are people of color. This document reflects a women of color perspective on the status of women, that *takes into consideration the complex intersections of other forms of discrimination* such as racism and classism, *that affect the human rights of women*.[58]

The delegates linked domestic and international social policy, highlighting the necessity of including US women of color in these discussions in part out of a sense of solidarity: US domestic policy influenced its international policies, which, they argued, affected similarly marginalized women elsewhere. Most importantly, the delegates insisted on an analysis that would examine women's experiences through a perspective that considered "the complex intersections of other forms of discrimination." Women were never "just" women who solely experience gender oppression.

Exchanging ideas in international settings and witnessing how women in other countries used a human rights frame to advocate for issues in their home country, however, was not necessarily a viable advocacy solution to the problems that social movements in the United States battled because social movements operate within a specific political context. Some US activists such as Linda Burnham felt that after Beijing and the development of the Beijing Platform for Action, the US government "did not take it too seriously."[59] Burnham had been active in the Third World Women's Alliance, organized delegations to the UN conference in Nairobi and Beijing, and later founded the Women of Color Resource Center in Oakland, California. Burnham also presented at earlier Sister-Song events, including a human rights training. Thus, she had experience with international organizing.

Despite the restrictive domestic political environment, the organizing that occurred leading up to the conference forged networks and offered inspiration that lasted after the conference. A SisterSong founder, Mary Chung Hayashi, reflected on the importance of the Beijing conference: "Just being around tens of thousands of women from all over the world. And it didn't matter that I was from California because there were so many Asians and there were so many African women, it just didn't matter. We just all are just one and just feeling like, 'Oh, I'm not a minority here. We're just all there because we care about women's issues.'"[60] Of course, opinions differed within and across delegations about what constituted a "women's issue." Still, like many minority women, Hayashi articulated that the conference reduced her feelings of isolation as she interacted with women of different countries and discovered that they could find common cause despite being from different national backgrounds.

According to one account, these events were critical for early reproductive justice activists: "Their participation in these international events produced significant shifts in their thinking about how to frame the demand for reproductive freedom for women of color in the United States. . . . They returned home determined to forge ahead in building a national movement of women of color for reproductive health that would, for the first time, incorporate the global human rights framework into their activism."[61] That determination, however, did not mean that people in other movements would recognize their efforts in this vein. When human rights activist Thomas wrote, "As an activist in this movement, I have often wondered why, when women from all over the world are increasingly incorporating international human rights into their work, U.S. activists are not," there was an assumption about who US activists were.[62] She makes some interesting points about the insularity of US activists relative to the global human rights movement, but her description of how women were not organizing around human rights favored a particular form of feminism, ignoring the organizing efforts of women of color. At the time of Thomas's writing, many US women had returned from the Beijing conference excited to "bring human rights home." Malika Dutt had already chronicled how some US women of color had engaged with the Beijing processes.[63] It was not a perfect engagement, if there can ever be such a thing. But there *was* organizing leading up to and continuing beyond Beijing. Thus, what Thomas identified was a lack of attention to human rights by *mainstream* US activists such as those affiliated with White, middle-class organizations. Meanwhile, US women of color were paying attention to human rights and what it could offer their organizing efforts in the United States.

4

Training the Trainers amidst Backlash

SisterSong's first conference program statement about the political context in which SisterSong developed could apply to contemporary emerging social movements: "The SisterSong Collective emerged at a crucial time in . . . herstory, a time when the civil rights and feminist movements were both experiencing critical backlash."[1] Even though a Democratic president, Bill Clinton, was in office when SisterSong was founded, the US political opportunity structure was not significantly more supportive of a broad-based human rights movement than it had been under Republican presidents. Debates about welfare have been part of the US discourse for centuries, albeit literally under different terms.[2] The Aid to Families with Dependent Children program (aka "welfare") offered aid in various forms to low-income families. In the 1970s, presidential candidate Ronald Reagan popularized the image of a "welfare queen," the term a Chicago-area newspaper used to describe a woman who was reported to have several aliases to collect benefits checks and drive numerous cars while receiving aid from the state.[3] While studies continued to show that numerically more Whites used welfare, Blacks and Latinos disproportionately utilized it.[4] After decades of "exposés" and misinformation, in the public discourse, welfare represented an entitlement program for lazy, scheming, poor Black and Latina women who did not want to work, instead preferring to become wealthy "queens" supposedly having many children to earn benefits, thereby taking advantage of (White) taxpayers' hard-earned money.

So presidential candidate Bill Clinton's promise to "end welfare as we know it" appealed to Republicans and more Democrats than cared to admit it. In 1996, one year after Beijing, and a year before the founding of SisterSong, Clinton made good on his promise. Welfare reform (or "deform," as some SisterSong leaders and other critics referred to it), heightened the discourses around poverty alleviation as a "handout."[5] The reforms resulted in the Temporary Assistance to Needy Families

(TANF) program, which amounted to a drastic reduction of one of the country's most vital economic support programs for low-income women and their children, the effects of which are still visible today. Major changes included a five-year lifetime limit on receipt of assistance, waiting periods for immigrants to receive assistance, "family caps" in which children born to a family already receiving welfare received drastically reduced or no benefits, and reduction in what counted as work activity. Specifically, attending school no longer counted as work activity. Thus, while social scientists produce studies showing that a person increasing his or her education was necessary to improve employment prospects, welfare recipients would not be able to do so with the assistance of the government. This shift to TANF is yet another example of what I demonstrated in prior chapters: the US government's relationship to broader human rights like economic rights had been forged decades earlier. The limited social movement opportunities to pressure the government necessitated a focusing on shifting cultural attitudes around human rights.

Welfare reform relied on images of Latinas and Black women as unrepentant reproducers. Black feminist theorist Patricia Hill Collins refers to these images as "controlling" because they represent dominant stereotypical images that shape the way people see Black women, historically and today.[6] These images are revised and updated in contemporary language, but at their base is a limited image that serves to demonize Black women's reproduction in particular, but not exclusively. While SisterSong was not specifically focused on welfare, a broader analysis of reproduction beyond abortion meant recognizing how policies differently affect people's reproduction and the contradictions embedded within policy. The same government that did not want to allocate budget funds for contraception or abortion for low-income people also did not want to support children of low-income people. Thus, developing an organization like SisterSong that would talk about support to have children and rights to parent was risky. Yet it was also a form of resisting the controlling images promoted by Clinton and his cronies.

Focusing on Women of Color Movement Sustainability

The seemingly "basic" concern of creating a sustainable movement for women of color that relied on a different way of understanding reproduction was not so basic if one keeps in mind that there is a long history of women in racial/ethnic movements having a role but finding their contributions interpreted by activists in other movements—and scholars—in narrow ways. Historically, White women participated in the US civil rights movements and the emerging New Left. Many people, Black and White alike, were inspired to join the civil rights movement after witnessing the persistence of groups like the NAACP and, later, the Student Nonviolence Coordinating Committee (SNCC). In these settings, movement participants realized the power—and cost—of collective action. Additionally, many White youth gained first-hand experience in community organizing and challenging racial inequality, an experience that encouraged them to develop their own organizations, such as Students for a Democratic Society (SDS).

Having learned social movement organizing skills in the South and working on poor people's campaigns, energetic students dreamed of a movement that challenged the status quo. In a key statement, the 1962 Port Huron Statement, Students for a Democratic Society advocated for participatory democracy alongside dismantling capitalism and racism. In their reflection on the statement forty years later, key leaders reminded readers of its origins: "The denial of dignity and the vote among blacks was a window into powerlessness in many forms. Young male students could be drafted to kill, but not to vote for peace candidates. A majority of Americans were denied any participation in decisions that were being made every day in their workplaces. Women were second class in every sphere of life. We agreed on a core principle: We demanded the right to vote as a first step toward a right to a voice and vote in all the decisions that affected our lives."[7] White women participated in these efforts, and a subset of activists developed an increasing feminist consciousness, objecting to serving as "movement housewives" who supported male activists through administrative work, cooking, and sexual relationships.[8] Two young White SNCC activists anonymously wrote a document entitled "SNCC Position Paper (Women in the Movement)," which a Black woman presented at a 1964 SNCC staff retreat. The position paper cited various incidents of sexism and claimed that, among other problems in SNCC, women were not given the same opportunities as men. When the paper began to circulate, some Black women who were garnering increasingly important roles in the movement felt "respected and admired for their strength and endurance" and expressed skepticism at the document's claims.[9]

Women of color had different roles in racial justice organization. While they did experience sexism, they also forged critical relationships. Again, in reexamining the US civil rights movement, Robnett shows that African American women were excluded from formal channels of leadership; thus they served as "bridge leaders" connecting with people emotionally in ways that facilitated their willingness to take the risk of joining the movement.[10] However, Black women's "bridge work," while vital, was less visible to outsiders, including researchers, the majority of whom saw leadership as men in movements saw it: a male endeavor.[11]

As change agents, Black women "use a wide range of strategies to 'change the realities' of their lives."[12] Yet, Springer identifies explicitly Black *feminist* organizing as "interstitial politics" that (1) occurs in everyday life and (2) occurs with consideration of intersecting effects of Black women's race, gender, and class.[13] Springer developed the idea of "interstitial politics" to encapsulate both types of activism in which Black women engaged. As Roth notes, Chicana activists of the 1960s and 1970s, in contrast to their Black counterparts, did not have some of the traditional spaces of organizing available, such as historically Black college campuses where they were in the racial majority.[14] Still, a vibrant set of activisms emerged on and off campuses in which Chicanas argued for Chicano liberation, cultural pride, remaking of the ideal of family to include recognition of women's contributions, and reproductive control, among other demands.[15]

As commitments have waned and various organizations have disappeared, activists and scholars have forgotten or ignored these histories. Women of color had been developing a movement preceded by prior projects, coalitions, initiatives, and the like. None of these had the sustainability of the mainstream reproductive rights movement that was dominated by the "big four" women's organizations: Feminist Majority Foundation, NARAL Pro-Choice America, National Organization for Women, and Planned Parenthood. Again, women of color of all racial backgrounds had been members of these organizations and in some cases, such as Planned Parenthood, even held leadership positions. Still, as Ferree noted in her study on abortion politics, which included interviews with the "big four" in the late 1990s, "As these organizational spokespeople admit, expanding the concept of reproductive rights is not today what the mainstream movement is seeking to achieve."[16] Rather, they were trying to engage with the hegemonic ideas of the discursive opportunity structure, which lent itself to a continued emphasis on reproductive rights and abortion as a choice. This required downplaying other needs and concerns, including the right to have children and the right to parent, which women of color raised in various terms.

Thus, it is not surprising that the idea of creating a sustainable movement came up continually in organizational documents, dominating other discussions. The mere existence of SisterSong was, according to one founder, a "ground breaking project that promises to make waves in the sea of complacency and neglect." The mainstream women's movement—and many in the public—were complacent about women of color improving their health. The needs of women of color were neglected, as confirmed from many quarters. Thus, even if mainstream women's organizations were going to pay attention to minority women, when it came to Black women, Ross insisted that "even with the best will in the world, white women will never represent the authenticity, authority, and uniqueness of African American women's experiences."[17] Thus, whether the focus was Black women, Chicanas, Latinas, Asian women, or Native women, the women themselves needed to be part of the discussion.

Just as Black women could not always fully assume solidarity, neither could Latinas, Asian/Pacific Islanders, or Indigenous women. Thus, to move forward required a continued commitment to movement sustainability. This was the type of work that, Springer reminds us, was articulated by Frances Beal: "'To die for the revolution is a one-shot deal; to live for the revolution means taking on the more difficult commitment of changing our day-to-day life patterns.'"[18] Changing patterns also meant understanding the nuances of different racial communities. In early Black women's organization, while there were initial assumptions of unity among Black feminists, they "discovered cleavages based on their inattention to class and sexual orientation as shapers of the parameters of black women's oppression."[19] Many minority-specific (social movement) organizations had emerged and ceased, so an organization that could sustain a movement base remained a priority.

Growing Pains in Claiming Human Rights for Women of Color

This section takes us into use of a human rights framework in the development of the coalition in its early stages. In it we find discussions of human rights as being relevant and needed and emerging *from* women of color–ness—from the embodied experiences of structural inequality. For example, I consider human rights trainings the early founders received and gave. In these early years we can see the development of the tension between the human rights perspective serving as a motivation for reproductive justice versus the human rights perspective as a strategy for promoting reproductive justice. Using the human rights frame as a motivation makes it a core, central, and continual goal in and of itself whereas the latter makes it present but in service of reproductive justice. If the human rights framework was the *motivation*, then reproductive justice could not exist without it. If it was a *strategy*, then it was one possible way of many to achieve reproductive justice.

An early SisterSong mission statement (1999) totaled three sentences:

> The SisterSong Women of Color Reproductive Health Collective is made up of local, regional and national grassroots organizations representing four primary ethnic populations/indigenous nations in the United States: Native American/Indigenous, Black/African American, Latina/ Puerto Rican and Asian/Pacific Islander. The Collective was formed with the shared recognition that as women of color we have the right and responsibility to represent ourselves and our communities. Sister-Song is committed to educat[ing] women of color on Reproductive and Sexual Health and Rights and work[ing] towards the access of health services, information and resources that are culturally and linguistically appropriate through the *integration of the disciplines of community organizing, Self-Help and human rights education.*[20]

This mission emphasized the importance of self-representation as both a right and a responsibility. Its last sentence persisted through various iterations of the mission statement, including years when the mission expanded to be twice as long and later when it was condensed again.

At the start of the millennium, the collective engaged in a number of outward-facing activities. SisterSong leaders reflected on the collective's origins and progress in a coauthored article in a public health journal. The article highlighted the many issues SisterSong was trying to address: lack of understanding of the scope of the reproductive health issues women of color faced; lack of culturally relevant health education and interventions; inadequacy of traditional reproductive rights advocacy in which women of color's reproductive experiences were largely not considered or at least not to the degree that they wanted; and more. The article outlined the organizational structure of the SisterSong Project, as it was referred to at the time, specific concerns four ethnic/racial mini-communities identified for their respective members, and the approach to reproduction SisterSong was trying to promote. As a starting point, the article's introduction connected domestic (US) and international experiences: "There is a dialectical relationship between what happens to women of color in other countries and what is visited upon women of color in the United States: all of our human rights are restricted by a white supremacist structure that de-prioritizes our needs while exploiting our bodies for the reproduction and maintenance of the economic system."[21] That women of color had a common experience was presumed. Or, at least it was presumed that while globally women of color experienced different problems, the root of them was the same—White supremacist capitalism—and the strategy to maintain these problems was the same—restricting human rights.

The authors placed SisterSong within a larger, developing US movement for human rights that was "demanding that the United States be held accountable to the same human rights standards that are recognized around the world."[22] As a practical matter, recognition of rights and accountability to protection of those rights were two different, albeit interrelated, problems. Still, the authors insisted that SisterSong was doing something unique by drawing on human rights discourse. Further, it argued, the US government's rejection of the range of human rights made *it* the outlier. The demands that SisterSong and others were making were necessary and particularly useful for reproductive advocacy since "the United States lacks a sufficient legal framework that guarantees women of color safe and reliable access to health care; emphasis on individual civil and political rights neglects economic, social, and cultural human rights that address group or collective needs. In order to ensure appropriate treatment and access to health care, and to address the intersectional oppression matrix (class, race, gender) that affects women of color, a comprehensive human rights–based approach is necessary."[23] Ross and her coauthors argued that women of color *as a group* had different needs due to the multiple oppressions they experienced. Of course, "women of color" was a broad category with no end of diversity—a diversity that was at times conflated to make a rhetorical point. Still, underpinning SisterSong's worldview about movement necessity and success was the imperative to operate from an understanding that women always had a gender identity, a racial identity, and a class position.

Articles such as this one contributed to the growing story of Sister-Song for researchers, the primary audience of the journal, and potential movement participants. The fact that the article's introduction included discussion of international conferences was important, as was the claim that SisterSong "draws inspiration and tools from the international human rights movement."[24] The authors were continuing to set a foundation for their future activities, of which they intended to engage in many, as demonstrated by grant proposals and concept papers wherein they laid out the collective's continued aims.

In describing prior efforts at developing a women of color reproductive advocacy network, SisterSong noted, "These efforts, like those that preceded them, failed not because of the lack of commitment, but because of the lack of resources. But they demonstrated that women of color must *develop an active reproductive and sexual health movement that is global,* and that helps us come together in a collaborative effort to address the lack of just choices for women in our communities."[25] In other places, founders have said that lack of resources was a problem, but a larger issue was that women of color were pulled in too many directions regarding their movement "loyalty" while also trying to create their own space.

That SisterSong's reach would ideally be global was emphasized in one of the concept paper's listed aims: "Policy that is developed and implemented as a result of this Project will have local, state, national and international impact."[26] This was an ambitious goal. Specific programs could have a broad reach through travel or even technology. However, policymaking at even the local level is arduous, let alone the global level, which includes, among other things, governments negotiating with each other and nongovernmental organizations trying to influence the process. Still, this statement shows the bold vision embedded in the aims of the collective, which was still gaining its footing.

The section on "future goals" began by discussing the relationship between health and human rights: "By increasing the awareness of women of color about threats to their health and by increasing their understanding of their human rights, we effect social change. Social change is the Collective's primary objective for the next phase of the SisterSong project."[27] As it looked to the future, SisterSong saw raising the consciousness of women *beyond* the collective as a primary tactic for change making. A handwritten note in red pen on the concept paper remarks, "Must reflect growth—what is new is reaching out to other mvts [movements] using the health rights framework."[28] This showed founders' awareness of the unusualness of using human rights framing.

As SisterSong retooled its organizational structure, the new Management Circle would, among other activities, "Ensure Self-Help and Human Rights Framework [Are] Operationalized at every level."[29] Exactly what counted as operationalization was not clear, nor were the consequences for missing the mark. In discussing expanding collective membership through the mini-community structure, attendees brainstormed three items. On the first two items, attendees were clear that the next set of organizations to join the collective needed to "serve women of color" and "have a reproductive rights agenda." However, the third criterion was less clear: "(Progressive? Women's human rights perspective) Agrees with principles of unity."[30] There was a question of whether the organizations needed to be "progressive," which was tentatively connected to emphasizing women's human rights. I note "tentatively" because the phrases were included in parentheses, unlike the other items. Further, the question mark indicates tentativeness on the part of some people at the meeting.

Hence, it seems that there was again a tension between using the human rights perspective as a frame or an intentional strategy or both. So, in some spaces, an idea being lauded as a critical aspect of reproductive justice—human rights—was inconsistently discussed as a requirement for participation in a collective that had at its core the goal of promoting reproductive justice. The meeting did produce concrete items, including the first Principles of Unity document. Three small groups brainstormed many values, including "Human rights and social justice activism" and "Work within a framework of self empowerment, human rights and respect of spiritual beliefs and practices of all women, including all indigenous traditional healing practices." Versions of these suggested items appeared in the later Principles of Unity, which organizational and individual members were required to agree to when formally joining the collective.

The People's Decade for Human Rights Education (PDHRE) spawned many efforts, including the Center for Human Rights Education (CHRE) in Atlanta, which opened in 1996. In its first year, CHRE claimed to have reached two thousand people, from community-based organizations to college campuses, through workshops and talks.[31] Its director, Loretta Ross, contributed an editorial to USA Today, a forum that would provide high visibility for any cause.[32] The editorial emphasized the need to ratify the Convention on the Elimination of All Forms of Discrimination Against Women (CEDAW).[33] Ross began with discussion of the court case about allowing women to enter the Virginia Military Institute. She claimed, "The entire controversy could have been avoided if Congress had passed the women's human rights treaty that has been languishing since 1980. Officially called the convention on Elimination of All Forms of Discrimination Against Women, the treaty would make these drawn-out court cases unnecessary. Women would not have to battle sex-discriminating institutions one by one, state by state and issue by issue. From welfare reform to sexual harassment, one treaty could cover it all."[34] Referring to Hillary Clinton's remarks at Beijing, Ross wondered if the Clinton administration would join the various US organizations that supported ratification of CEDAW. While the editorial offered an overly optimistic view of the effects a treaty would have on deeply entrenched sexism in the United States, it successfully linked a range of issues—occupational segregation, child care, violence, welfare rights, retirement, healthcare—and suggested how viewing these issues as linked was possible: through the lens of human rights. Ross was clearly a believer in the domestic human rights project and promoted human rights as a solution to many social problems.

Many SisterSong founders viewed attending international conferences as a way both to increase the visibility of women of color internationally and to gain new strategies for domestic activism. While UN conferences proved fruitful for visibility and strategy, there were other important settings. At an October 1997 SisterSong meeting, a discussion addressed the role of delegates to the Fourth International Congress on AIDS. Delegates had specific instructions: "Let other people of color know—our struggle is the same. . . . [B]ring back materials distributed by pharmaceutical companies, [e]xplain the invisibility of Asian[s] and Native Americans in the USA. . . . Take notes of how many women speakers versus the number of men speakers, [s]pot and [o]utreach to other women of color to build networks, [and] [r]eturn with information about how other groups are doing effective work." The role of the delegates was the first item on the agenda, which suggests that Sister-Song foregrounded the international networking in which the group was engaging.

The Ford Foundation sponsored a delegation to attend the Fourth Annual International Congress on AIDS in Asia and the Pacific Rim, which took place in Manila, Philippines, in October 1997. Four delegates, all of them involved in SisterSong, represented US women of color: Dázon Dixon Diallo of SisterLove Women's AIDS Project, Mary Chung of the National Asian Women's Health Organization, Luz Rodriguez of the Latina Roundtable on Health and Reproductive Rights, and Barbara Skytears Moore (Apache) of the Moon Lodge Native American Women's Outreach Project. According to an account in the newspaper, these delegates discussed "the modern day sex-slave trade of women throughout the world, sky-rocketing rates of HIV infection in Africa, and an epidemic of HPV in young girls throughout the world. The delegation returned to the emerging SisterSong Collective with a more global perspective of how human rights are intertwined with reproductive health and sexual rights of women of color, and how the grassroots sisterhood of activists in the United States is forever connected to the plight of women and girls of color throughout the world."[35] From this reflection, we learn the influence of an international conference. A select group of participants developed connections with other organizations, observed human rights education in an international setting, and thus formed a "more global perspective" on the domestic issues around which they were organizing. This reflection relied on essentialist ideas of sisterhood that presume commonality across gender, but added nuance by emphasizing that the sisterhood specifically contained both grassroots activists in the United States and all women of color elsewhere. Still, while the newspaper article does suggest a need to differentiate between advocacy approaches by women of color in the United States, the differentiation does not extend to the varied experience within the category of non-US women of color. The article presents a simultaneously hopeful and idealistic representation of the connections between minority women in the United States and elsewhere.

Dázon Dixon Diallo, a public health activist, had been organizing around HIV and noted the importance of the intersection between reproductive justice and HIV. When considering how the frameworks connected, she reflected, "The way I do describe the way the intersection between reproductive justice, and human rights looks like is just this. I really start with the human rights lens. Right? Because, first of all, everybody doesn't know where you want them to go when you say 'human rights,' right? People have their own notions of what that means, and most often, they're stuck on civil rights and poverty. They don't know what to do with that, they don't know how it's protected [laughs], but that's where people are." Her point was that people needed clarity on their right to have rights. She continued,

> It's almost like what happens on the computer now with Windows or with Mac, you know? You've got one window, and you can click on something and open up another window. . . . So if human rights is the operating system [laughs], right, and then you click on the RJ window and it opens up, and you can look at, for women with HIV, issues around equal access to abortion as a choice . . . but I also don't want to be discriminated against by people who want to force abortion on me as a choice because they don't believe in HIV-positive women's sexuality and ability to parent. . . . You would look at the level of insurance coverage or housing opportunities or job opportunities. All of these situations that present themselves that we know are required to have in place for folks to have equal opportunity with their reproductive health outcomes.[36]

With the human rights framework as an "operating system," it was to provide the basis for the reproductive justice movement and offer people different "windows" of analysis.

There were many aspects to developing a new women of color collaborative that would need to be addressed. At the March 1997 symposium, the agenda for a small group exercise had five broad areas, including "basic needs" and "leadership roles," both of which appear to be internally focused activities about the development of the SisterSong initiative. Under the area "level of awareness," one of the questions asked, "Are women of our communities able to relate the significance of their own well being to the issues of human rights?"[37] Leaders remained unsure what it could mean to engage their respective communities on these issues and how to help their constituents understand international human rights discourse as relevant to the domestic political sphere. At another meeting that fall, a group of about twenty representatives met. According to the notes, only one attendee identified anything related to human rights. In the description of her work, Pandora Singleton, an AIDS activist, reportedly said that she "offers HIV testing and provides counseling services of programs who support pro-life and human rights in women of color."[38] This is an interesting grouping of programs: pro-life and human rights. But it was not on everybody's mind, and the fact that "human rights" appears only once suggests that it was not everyone's motivation.

While there were still many details to figure out about the fledgling collective, there was substantial excitement. In an e-mail discussion about the evaluations from an October 1997 meeting, SisterSong's program officer at the Ford Foundation, Reena Marcelo, responded optimistically about the possibilities of SisterSong to bring together different perspectives:

> The more I think about the potentials of this aggrupation, the more excited I get. Like for example the exchange of resources and expertise across cultural groupings for skills and knowledge building in research, advocacy, service provision, community outreach and education. . . . [I]t would also help to demonstrate that work amongst different cultural groups can be beneficial to all, exciting, that differences can be assets as well in women's empowerment and community and development. Am I dreaming too much?!!! :] knock me on the head if it seems that I am![39]

Nevertheless, the collective's members still had much to learn. CHRE saw itself as doing innovative work: "pioneering ground-breaking human rights education" by "reaching directly into diverse communities of activists who work on all social justice issues."[40] That activists themselves needed training on human rights was assumed. This education was a vital part of revolutionary domestication of the human rights agenda: "Human rights education also links international treaties to local issues, moving the prosaic words of treaties into meaningful ways to take action." The use of "prosaic" indicates that the grant writer understood that for many audiences the government documents merely appeared like dry government language. Of course, the words themselves hide histories of conflict between governments and the possibilities of future visions for activists.

CHRE focused on learning from women globally while sharing points of commonality. Its Odyssey Project offers an illustrative example. The project, the full name of which was Women's Health 2001: A Human Rights Odyssey, aimed to connect US activists with international human rights activists:

> The Center for Human Rights Education has already begun a program called the Odyssey Project that educates women activists, community members and organizers in HIV/AIDS and women's human rights. It targets women of color in the southern region of the U.S. and connects them with communities of women in developing countries all over the globe. International women's human rights and health educators share their experiences with the U.S. women, and promote the development and actions of their struggling organizations. This new collective identifies all communities of women of color as the developing world inside the U.S. and will intentionally respond to organizations from all over.[41]

Again, these words demonstrate both an excitement about learning from women *outside* the United States and an articulation of similarity of experience with these women. The belief that US minority women experienced solidarity with women elsewhere was emphasized through designation of both groups of women as "developing." That said, CHRE's emphasis was on Black women, as illustrated by its aim both to "do outreach to *other* especially black women's organizations and communities,"[42] presenting at events such as the International Black Women's Cross-Cultural Institute in Johannesburg and Struggles of Black Men and Women in Latin America, and to situate itself within SisterSong's African American mini-community.

In providing feedback on the grant proposal, the Ford Foundation asked for a revised document that included, among other changes, integration of answers to two questions: "Can you include in the proposal a description of CHRE strategies for changing U.S. policies to ratify the HR [human rights] treaty, and the role that these NGOs will play in implementing this strategy? Also, include a discussion of the barriers to ratification of this treaty that you will foresee."[43] These two questions were deceptively simple and highlight the utopian vision the proposal represented. First, it is hard to imagine how CHRE—or any organization—could on its own change US policies. Second, even if there were changes in US policies, that would not necessarily lead to ratification of treaties. US policies had changed many times, but this was not, for various reasons, with an eye toward what was happening at the UN. Finally, the list of barriers to ratification could be so numerous as to take up the whole proposal. And again, for many of these barriers, overcoming them would be well beyond the scope of CHRE's work or that of any one organization. Thus, while the genre of grant proposal writing is one that encourages applicants to present an attractive, albeit usually unreachable, set of goals their organization aims to achieve, these three comments were reminding the author to consider reality.

In applying to the Ford Foundation, CHRE identified the need for capacity-building funds for the many ways they could help, from needs assessment to grant writing. "Human rights" fell in the middle of the capacity-building list. Yet, the proposal suggested that the CHRE, as a member of the African American mini-community, receive twenty-five thousand dollars of the grant "to conduct human rights education and advocacy workshops and programs for groups involved in SisterSong, as well as for groups affiliated with the SisterSong network. This program would provide greater awareness of women's human rights and would promote women's rights within the context of reproductive health and RTIs [reproductive tract infections] among women of color."[44] In this same grant, only three of sixteen organizations referenced "human rights" in their activities: two from the African American community (CHRE and Project Azuka, Pandora Singleton's organization); and one from the Latin American community (Fundacion AIDS de Puerto

Rico Inc., which housed the program Grupo de Derechos Reproductivos).[45] CHRE and Grupo referenced human rights several times. Thus, while human rights were central for some collective members, the idea was not on the radar for most of the other organizations, at least not in those terms. On one hand, this suggests that member organizations did not prioritize human rights. On the other hand, it showed the need for CHRE to conduct educational sessions for the broader collective membership.

CHRE envisioned its work having a broad impact: "CHRE can strengthen and inform the Women's Reproductive Health movement in its experience with women's human rights and reproductive health and education and its networking capacity."[46] Further, it would encourage participation in celebrations of the Universal Declaration of Human Rights, which indicates a clear idea of having people connect human rights to the UN. This was not necessarily a common vision of women of color organizations. As CHRE was noting, it had a unique role to fill *because* of its interest in human rights in the United States. Therefore, using an anomalous approach would mean taking on an uphill battle.

CHRE was a small organization that, at times, operated primarily from Ross's home with her financial support, which she provided by risking her own credit.[47] While this is common for grassroots organizations, it is a reminder of the personal dedication grassroots activists hold for their causes—much like entrepreneurs who invest their personal resources to start a business. With limited financial resources, CHRE was connecting with both local and international movements. The sponsorship of and connection to SisterSong were critical for integration of human rights discourse.

The clarity of CHRE's plans in its concept paper stands in contrast to some of the other concept papers. For example, the Latina Roundtable concept paper was divided into three years of activities. Year 1 was developing capacity such as a board and securing volunteers, and year 2 was programming on reproductive health and position papers. Only in year 3 was there reference to human rights in the plan to "conduct an organizational training workshop for other grassroots organizations in the development of non-profit advocacy initiatives, reproductive health and rights issues as [they pertain] to their respective missions and human rights."[48] With regard to planning, this is a realistic accounting of the time it takes to develop an initiative. Yet it is notable that human rights training did not appear as a priority in the first year.

Human Rights: A Priority among Many

Even though several SisterSong founders articulated a desire to develop a movement for reproductive justice based on a human rights frame, there were still issues to resolve, such as the founders' own lack of understanding of human rights. After organizing the first official SisterSong meeting in Dallas in 1998, CHRE also provided human rights training at it.[49] The goals were several, including "to learn about women's human rights and their relevance to the lives of women of color in the U.S."[50] At the collective's first training in 1998, one of the three topics for discussion was human rights, so it was formally on the agenda with a three-hour session titled "Human Rights Education." The three listed objectives for the CHRE-sponsored training were as follows:

Objective 1—Learn the basics about human rights including the Universal Declaration of Human Rights and other international documents/ instruments that can be used effectively in the integration of RTIs [reproductive tract infections] and Self-Help into the Collective.

Objective 2—Determine the universality, indivisiveness, and interconnectedness of political, economic, social and cultural rights within the context of their influence on RTIs and women's reproductive health needs.

Objective 3—Develop and adopt a SisterSong collective statement on women's rights as human rights with particular emphasis on reproductive health and RTIs.[51]

The first objective illustrates an example of revolutionary domestication in that it drew on specific United Nations documents to show the relevance of international human rights discourse for domestic political advocacy. The second objective challenged the public (state) and private (domestic) binary by making clear that all of these rights were connected to the very personal, usually private, problem of reproductive tract infections.

Any one of these objectives would be a major undertaking, so this was a packed agenda for a few hours, particularly when founding members were still learning about human rights themselves. In evaluating the meeting, Luz Rodriguez, one of the founders, felt that the portion of the training on human rights "was too brief to thoughtfully make the connections as I may be one of those women who doesn't know *all* of her rights yet."[52] Receiving information about human rights and talking through the ideas for a few hours was not enough for Rodriguez to feel comfortable with her understanding of human rights. Her observation is particularly interesting considering that she was one of the four delegates that the Ford Foundation had sponsored to attend the Manila conference the year prior and, therefore, had more exposure to human rights discourse than many of the other attendees. Rodriguez continued: "Perhaps we were too ambitious to attempt 3 areas of training in one. Further trainings such as this one should allow generous time for each area. It occurs to me that the Human Rights Trainings will be on-going—so should the self-help and RTIs just like the Tele-comm & Fiscal. Just a reflection on our visioning, and how we see things better once we begin to manifest the vision. Perhaps supplemental resources can be obtained for on-going training at the 16 sites."[53] The need for ongoing discussion about core ideas is not unique to SisterSong.

As sociologist Jessica Taft notes in her study of girls' activism, movements engage in numerous forms of political education. Education includes basic knowledge construction, which relies on the assumption that providing potential supporters with information leads them to change their minds; feeling production, which relies on the assumption that producing feelings in potential supporters spurs them to action; and ongoing process, which relies on the assumption that education happens in many arenas.[54] Rodriguez's reflection highlights how human rights education was not a one- or even two-time experience. Rather, it was a lengthy process that was occurring among many other commitments and pressures.

As with any movement, there are multiple narratives. In my interviews with founders and people who attended early SisterSong meetings, there were different ideas about the importance of human rights. In my interview with Latonya Slack, who was based in California, she reflected on how the concept of human rights influenced her organization's work with Black women.

Well, definitely, you mention human rights and human rights model. That wasn't, early on, I mean it wasn't, you know, initially I don't remember us talking about, but somewhere, you know, in those first—, the first four years I would say, we got a training on the human rights model and how that human rights work was used in international communities, European, what the tenets were of that model, and then how it could be adopted in the United States. And so that was also a framework that we talked about and included it in each of our gatherings. You know, discussions about this and ways to implement it and use it. And in that instance, I do remember Loretta Ross being one of the primary advocates of this human rights model. But it was influential to us as a statewide organization.[55]

Here, one founder described what she saw as a positive experience of exposure to human rights. While at first, she says the human rights frame was not "initially" included, she recalls that there *was* a training. She also says the training included an "international" element to it ("European"). Then she considers various instances of exposure in the early years of SisterSong. Further, she describes the framework being useful in later work upon which her Black women's health organization embarked. I conducted her interview more than a decade after the training; thus the fact that she could remember that there had been a training despite the many intervening years indicates that it made some type of lasting impression.

However, the consistent discussion of human rights in SisterSong's early years does not mean there was complete allegiance to this concept serving as an organizing frame. In one interview, Sonya, a Latina woman who helped found SisterSong, provided an alternative perspective. She felt that the idea of human rights was new to many people embarking on founding the collective in the mid-1990s. When considering the founding of SisterSong, Sonya expressed, "CEDAW and all that stuff. Okay, so, so I think that was part of, while it [SisterSong] came into being, it also created tension because I would say, you know, even internally in the group there was no democratization of the human rights framework." Any scholar of movements or movement participant would not be surprised to hear about "tensions," as these are a common part of movement development. However, even if there was not an actual "tension," as Sonya described it, she points to a lack of "democratization."

This can be taken several ways. The first interpretation is that there was simply a lack of understanding about human rights among the early collective members. As she explains, "But part of the problem of that whole language [of human rights] was that it was really a language of estrangement, and it was an academic sort of foreign language, I think, even to some of the other members of the collective. . . . In a domestic level, we're dealing more with like civil rights language." Sonya highlighted a few challenges with "human rights" that she did not believe were limited to her, specifically that the language appeared as "foreign" and international. She later identified human rights with an "international body." Yet, human rights appeared abnormal since this was a concept used in international arenas. Moreover, part of the foreignness came from the appearance as *academic*, or in other words, not practical.

It is this challenge that SisterSong founders had to consider in building their own base. This points to a larger challenge of promoting human rights more broadly. Further, other narratives were still present. For example, some foundation funders focused on public health frameworks of disease prevention that emphasized education around reproductive tract infections, as they were called then. Sonya's response illustrated why there would be a need for revolutionary domestication that constructs international human rights discourse as relevant for the domestic political sphere. Moreover, a second interpretation of Sonya's comment about democratization is that there was not widespread *participation* in the decision-making process about human rights being core to the collective's continued development. Sonya further reflected, "Publicly it's easy because you can see all the [SisterSong] documents . . . and you'll see that a large part of it is about that human rights framework. And I'm not saying that's not important: it is. I'm just saying that I don't think it was a shared—that there wasn't necessarily total consensus on that being sort of the main driver." Her comment identified a different issue than lack of knowledge: a lack of *will*.

Another interviewee, "Jayne," an Asian/Pacific Islander organizer, also challenged the SisterSong narrative about the importance of international conferences in its development. She felt that since many people did not have the opportunity to attend those conferences, they did not hold as important a role for later core members in committing to Sister-Song's goal of broadening understanding and advocacy around reproduction to include rights to have children and rights to parent. Jayne saw the connection to human rights as resulting from the particularities of reproductive activism at the time:

> They felt like "reproductive justice"—it was a palatable form for Americans to talk about the human rights issues. And at the same time there were a lot of grassroots, indigenous kind of culture and people that sort of grassroots, indigenous groups who started doing reproductive rights work in a very different way that was much more sort of community-centered, was much more about empowerment and organizing. I think like ACRJ [Asian Communities for Reproductive Justice, now Forward Together] is one of those groups or, you know, CLRJ [California Latinas for Reproductive Justice]. And so that there was the emergence of reproductive justice movement that extends from the bottom up, as opposed to some international groups in the U.S. And so, in some ways, within the reproductive justice movement is this perfect storm of international human rights work coming to the United States and this very kind of grassroots, inundated women of color–led work, you know, creating a new paradigm has come together to form this very broad umbrella called reproductive justice. And SisterSong plays one role in that, but there are many others.[56]

While the personal biographies of movement founders influenced SisterSong's development, Jayne contested the importance of certain events, focusing instead on a collective story of emergence.[57] Intracoalition skepticism about the human rights framework certainly existed. Formally, however, the SisterSong coalition embraced it.

With the extrinsic and intrinsic problems of organizing using a human rights framework, we come back to the initial puzzle of why SisterSong founders chose to use that framework for US-based advocacy. While at SisterSong's 2009 membership meeting in Washington, DC, I conducted a number of interviews. One was with Luz Rodriguez, a Latina SisterSong founder and long-time board treasurer whom some people referred to as "Mama Luz."[58] She explained what she remembered as the power of a human rights frame in those early years: "[T]he common thread that every woman from all these different nations and ethnic backgrounds found was that we all had a history of sterilization abuse, and we all had a history of human rights violation. So it wasn't just Puerto Rican women [but also] Black women from their history, Native women from their history, Asian women from their history, and that fueled SisterSong [bringing palm together, interlacing fingers, and laughing]. That bonded [us], that was like doing a glue gun."[59]

While Rodriguez told me this in a personal interview, she repeated a version of this story at various public SisterSong events. The story reiterates the idea that the remedy to the founders' ancestral, and in some cases, personal, histories of reproductive violation were *only* understandable through a human rights frame. These experiences were unintelligible when "read" through arguments about "choice."

As had been proposed in grants, there were indeed more human rights trainings. Canción Latina, the name for the Latino mini-community, received a full-day training from CHRE in May 2000.[60] The training mixed presentations by CHRE staff and discussion (see table 4.1). Before lunch, the sessions offered introductions to human rights (e.g., "What I know about Human rights"). An hour was dedicated to a discussion of the Universal Declaration of Human Rights. The agenda included handwritten modifications.

Table 4.1. Agenda for Canción Latina Training by CHRE (How to Use Human Rights in Your Organizing Efforts)

Training		
9:30–9:45	Pre-test: What I know about Human rights	Group Discussion
9:45–10:30	Introduction: My Life and Human Rights	Group Discussion
10:30–11:00	Planning the Day: What I want to Learn and Share	Group Discussion
11:00–12:00	Universal Declaration of Human Rights	CHRE Staff
*Military presence in Puerto Rico [hand-written note: In response to suggestion by Haydee @ Casa Atabex Aché]		
12:30–1:30	Lunch break [handwritten note: Hotel restaurant]	
1:30–3:00	Reproductive Rights and Human Rights	CHRE Staff
3:00–3:45	Using Human Rights	CHRE Staff
Taking Action: Using the Human Rights Framework		
3:45–4:00	Post-Test: What I Learned	
*Haydee Has Materials & a video that she is interested in showing		

CHRE, "How to Use Human Rights in Your Organizing Efforts" Canción Latina SisterSong Annual Meeting May 31, 2000, SisterSong files, Atlanta, GA.

This as an example of *revolutionary domestication* in which international human rights discourse was relevant to the domestic political sphere.[61] On the surface, the way military presence in Puerto Rico fit into a discussion on reproductive rights might not be clear. But the fact that it appeared on the agenda at the request of a member organization demonstrated the collective's process and the links members made between different issues. Further, that a day-long discussion dedicated to examining how human rights connected to reproductive rights could accommodate a discussion of militarism speaks to the expansiveness of the collective's vision and its objective to represent a range of women of color perspectives. "Women of color" was itself a diverse category—women of color were the same in their overall difference from White people, but different within the category, requiring attending to different manifestations of power, in this case how the nation produced neocolonial relationships.[62] Historically, the US state had inserted itself in the private lives of women, so women had to continue to make the connections about how national-level institutions with a global reach, such as the US military, affected women's reproductive health, a "private" matter. Challenging the public/private binary that the mainstream reproductive rights movement commonly upheld was another feature of revolutionary domestication.

The Latina mini-community continued to connect with their Puerto Rican counterparts through both education and in-person contact. Notes on a discussion of who would represent the mini-communities at a December 2000 conference on sexually transmitted diseases included a reminder that "the Latina mini-community will be in Puerto Rico during this time working on issues related to the United States' continued use and destruction of Vieques and its impact on the reproductive health of women in Vieques."[63] This referred to a history of medical experimentation on the island. In the 1950s, the Puerto Rican territory, responding both to US government pressure and desires to become more economically competitive, began a number of social engineering programs. Besides a widespread sterilization program that the Puerto Rican government implemented to make women workers more reliable, it also implemented a favorable tax structure to attract US mainland companies, which continues today.[64] Puerto Rico also served as a primary testing site for early oral contraceptives, such as the pill that Dr. Gregory

Pincus developed with the financial support of philanthropist Katharine McCormack and birth control advocate Margaret Sanger. Hundreds of Puerto Rican women eagerly took the experimental treatment with little information. The pill proved effective at preventing pregnancy. Yet, when Puerto Rican women complained of side effects, medical staff downplayed the complaints or ignored them outright. With the efficacy of the new pill documented, Pincus moved forward in development and the pill went into production, providing a financial boon to its producer, Searle, and mainland women of all races some degree of sexual freedom. However, what is now known as "the Pill" came at a cost—namely, the health of many Puerto Rican women.[65]

While Puerto Rican women are somewhat familiar with this history and its continuing effects, it remains largely unknown to many other oral contraceptive users. The Latina mini-community's trip offered yet another reminder that even within the United States, women of color had several "domestic" spheres in which they were embedded. For some women of color, that sphere included the US territory that remained economically and politically tied to the mainland. Thus, geopolitical boundaries affected SisterSong members differently and in this way offered another reason why a narrow view of reproduction that focused solely on the concerns of White middle-class women—or US women of any race—lacked appeal. Sexual freedom for some women had come at a cost to other women, a history that movement founders could not ignore and worked to avoid having repeated.

CHRE conducted human rights trainings for some of the mini-communities, like Canción Latina. Further, CHRE engaged in a CEDAW training as part of a national effort to strategize around ratification of CEDAW.[66] CHRE continued to educate other SisterSong members through providing information on development in human rights internationally, such as giving out copies of international-focused academic journals.[67] CHRE staff joined SisterSong member organization Sister-Love in South Africa in conducting human rights training.

The minutes from a January 2002 meeting showed both the way SisterSong was intentionally working to integrate the human rights frame into its efforts and the negotiation around how much the collective could require potential new members to do so. The first section, "What have we done," listed four items. The second, "Make international connections (Cuba, Puerto Rico/Vieques, South Africa, Jamaica, Canada)," again showed the continued efforts in the growing collective to exchange ideas with organizations/practitioners across borders. The third item noted that SisterSong "took RTI agenda and broadened it into Sexual/ Reproductive Rights Human Rights Framework." This referred to the funders' initial interest in supporting initiatives that had a disease-focused model.[68] It is important to remember that at the time dominant disease prevention models emphasized getting people to change their individual behavior. That SisterSong had been able to make the case that preventing disease required talking about the *context* of the disease was an important victory. This was SisterSong's way of revolutionary domestication—shifting mindsets to prime them for further advocacy.

There were a limited number of allies trying to do this work with reproduction in mind. Again, harkening back to Roskos's point, in comparison to international counterparts, there did not appear to be as vibrant a US women's movement addressing human rights.[69] Yet, there were some groups still trying to link US activism to human rights.

Finding Allies and Funding a "Revolution of the Mind"

This section traces a sampling of the many interconnections, discussions, and sharing of ideas across sectors. Over many years, the Institute for Women and Ethnic Studies (IWES) held a series of workshops with various stakeholders that focused on women of color and reproductive technology. The stakeholders included grassroots activists, medical professionals, and even representatives of pharmaceutical companies. Founded in 1993, IWES was a New Orleans nonprofit focused on community health. Out of the workshops came the Reproductive Bill of Rights, which was also referred to more specifically as the Reproductive Health Bill of Rights for Women of Color. A second version of the bill was released in 2001. Dr. Denese Shervington, one of the official 1994 Cairo women of color delegates to the UN conference on Women, Population, and Development, was connected to IWES. Two of the early participants in developing SisterSong, Charon Asetoyer of the Native American Women's Health Education Resource Center and Luz Alvarez Martinez of the National Latina Health Organization, participated in the IWES workshops. Other important intellectual figures, such as

Black feminist legal scholar Dorothy Roberts and feminist philosopher and White ally Marlene Gerber Fried, participated in the workshops as well.[70]

The Reproductive Health Bill of Rights for Women of Color was a colorful pamphlet and a rare comprehensive document in that it included the history of various conferences and workshops, the text of the bill, and a list of workshop attendees. The first part of the pamphlet began with a multiparagraph purpose statement. It read, "All people are born free and equal with dignity and rights as set forth in the Universal Declaration of Human Rights. Historically, women of color across nations, cultures and ethnic groups have been subject to racist exploitation, discrimination and abuse. Manipulative, coercive and punitive health policies and practices deprive women of color of their fundamental human rights and dignity."[71] Beginning with the UDHR shows how human rights was of even greater importance than highlighting the commonality of experiences for women of color, which, the document later specified, included "indigenous women and all other women who are discriminated against due to categorization within a particular racial or ethnic group."[72]

The bill itself started with a preamble, much like the US Bill of Rights, and referenced international conferences. The document drew on international concepts while also using the language of the US legal system as its basis. The document noted that it "endorses the principles and plans of the International Conference on Population and Development in Cairo and the Fourth World Conference on Women in Beijing. This Bill of Rights is the cornerstone of a global partnership that works to ensure that all women, particularly women of color, have access to appropriate health care services, information, and education so that they can make informed choices for attainment of the highest standards of sexual and reproductive health."[73] After the bill came the explanatory "background and history" section. In explaining the process of moving from the first to the second version, the brochure noted that feedback on the first version included the need to address indigenous women's concerns. Five items the workshop participants had agreed upon were included as well. The second to last item is particularly telling: "Women of color should insist that reproduction be seen as an issue of social justice, demanding equality among groups and not solely on the narrow issue of individual rights, especially those enjoyed primarily by privileged women."[74] Again we can appreciate the emphasis on paying attention to reproduction occurring within context. The reference to "individual rights" and "privileged women" subtly alluded to the individual right to abortion on which White women of the mainstream reproductive health and rights movement focused. Groups like National Latina Institute for Reproductive Health, which was involved with SisterSong's founding, endorsed the final document.

US activists convened in 1999 and 2002 to discuss US human rights organizing. From these two meetings came the idea for the US Human Rights Network. Two SisterSong founders, Dázon Dixon Diallo and Loretta Ross, both participated in the July 2002 Leadership Summit on Human Rights in the United States. In the resulting report, *Something Inside So Strong: A Resource Guide on Human Rights in the United States*, the authors reflected on the limitations of the civil rights framework.[75] They wrote, "Traditionally, U.S. activists have attacked these problems using the laws, media and other means available to them domestically. Most Americans know that they have certain rights that are enshrined in the Constitution and federal and state laws. There is an increasing awareness, however, that these domestic protections are not enough. The courts are increasingly conservative and hostile to civil and economic rights."[76] In a context in which the US government was engaging in restrictive domestication, activists were realizing that they needed to consider a different approach than the traditional legal-centered model.

The report offered a human rights framework as a *supplement* to create social change, providing "activists an additional rights vision, framework and set of tools to use in their struggles for justice in the United States. These are not meant to replace existing laws and strategies, but to bolster them and provide new avenues of activism. This framework and tools, rooted in the concept of 'human rights,' are not new. Their precursors are evident in the abolitionist movement."[77] The report authors pointed to a past injustice—slavery—as an example of an issue that lent itself to human rights advocacy. Here is an example of different understandings of human rights. In considering the origin of the concept of human rights, it is possible to understand this concept as having its origin from elsewhere, such as the United Nations. In contrast, it is also possible to understand the human rights framework as already existing in the United States and therefore from the United States. The former approach leads to connecting the concept of human rights with the "foreign," whereas the latter approach leads to connecting it with the familiar.

The report's general section on "discrimination" gave examples of Supreme Court cases that referenced international human rights law. Again, reiterating the hostile political environment and the potential of a human rights frame to combat it, the authors observed, "The current domestic climate in the United States is characterized by a sustained attack on the legal and political framework that combats discrimination and inequality in this country. Civil rights and remedies are being systematically curtailed by all three branches of a hostile and increasingly conservative federal government. By contrast, the human rights framework defines discrimination as an issue of substantive, rather than solely legal inequality, and thus may positively influence the debate on issues such as affirmative action and drug sentencing."[78] Essentially, the authors were saying that "human rights" was about more than legal inequality; it was also about practical inequality. They were arguing that human rights could address "the gap" that sociolegal scholars have identified as being the difference between law on the books and law in practice. The authors were alluding to the limitations of the civil rights frame, which is traditionally understood as ensuring nondiscrimination for protected classes.

The report was written in SisterSong's earlier years, which coincided with George W. Bush's first term as president. Under him, the hostile conditions described in the report would continue to hold. In fact, as the Bush administration continued to respond to the terrorist attack on the World Trade Center in 2001, formal law became a tool able to be wielded even more forcefully against activists. Citizens could not rely on basic liberties being protected, as the US was in what philosophers such as Agamben have identified as a perpetual "state of exception" that permitted state power to extend beyond the rule of law.[79] Thus, for activists to demand that the US government go beyond formal equality to promote conditions of thriving, and base a movement on that demand, was indeed revolutionary.

In the realm of funding, social movements have long been concerned about resources and the role of foundations in shaping their movements. Yet, funding paid people's salaries, bought materials for events, and even got people to events. While the relationship between human rights and reproductive justice on the surface was not connected to funding, at its core there were connections. So, talking about reproductive justice and human rights created a niche for SisterSong—there were SMOs talking about reproductive issues and SMOs talking about human rights, but linking the two for the purposes of action in the United States was novel.

SisterSong's initial funding had come from the Ford Foundation, which had a prior history of funding human rights work abroad. Amid the effort to create a sustainable movement for and of women of color in the United States while maintaining some type of connection—ideologically and physically—with women of color outside the United States was the need for a range of resources. SisterSong benefitted from philanthropy efforts to "bring human rights home." Some major funders, particularly the Ford Foundation, began a concerted effort to fund US-based projects engaging with human rights. Ford's *Close to Home* report highlighted a handful of these efforts that it funded.[80] A few assumptions underlie the invoking of "home." First, it identifies the United States as home. Second, it makes clear that this is an *active, continuing* process. Third, bringing human rights "home" fits into the narrative of human rights advocacy being from elsewhere. Finally, the idea also connotes *emphasizing* human rights, as in to "bring the point home." Various advocates have struggled to make the United States feel like home, where historical oppression of their communities made clear that they were not welcome. The idea of "bringing" is active work, so "human rights" can be a strategy to create home with tools from elsewhere. Interestingly, this does reinforce the idea that human rights is an idea from *outside* to be brought in, which plays into the public/private binary.

An example of a Ford activity was its Reproductive Health Affinity Group, which created a Human Rights and Sexuality and Reproductive Health Committee (HR & SRCH) that met throughout 2002. In its initial incarnation, the HR & SRHC aimed "to advance conceptualization/content of sexual rights and reproductive rights from a comprehensive human rights approach" so as "to advance thinking on the links between the reproductive health and human rights communities."[81] The cases attendees would analyze drew from "real-life situations" globally. The US case for attendees to analyze profiled "Peggy," a fictitious woman, who seemed to have faced almost every single obstacle possible in life. She is a homeless Guyanese immigrant formerly employed as a maid, addicted to drugs, who was not a US citizen and had "delivered an extremely premature and crack-addicted baby girl." In the scenario, Peggy meets a social worker who also happens to be of Guyanese descent and formerly homeless; the social worker begins to help Peggy rebuild her life.[82].

The point of the initial HR & SRCH meeting was to focus on commonalities, but the Ford Foundation found the approaches so irreconcilable that it created separate documents for the two groups in attendance: public health experts and human rights experts. Whereas sexual and reproductive health was in the realm of public health, human rights advocacy occurred in a different sphere. The expert groups received the same cases to review, but were provided different questions to answer, "in order to capture the different ways that the public health and human rights fields conceptualize and address issues"; thus the wording differed slightly for each group of experts.[83] Under "Actors/Institutions" the public health experts were to consider these questions: "Which actors/institutions are responsible for addressing this type of situation and determining the course of action? Do adequate institutions and procedures exist to address the situation described through a public health approach, and if not, how might these challenges be met?" The human rights experts were to consider a similar set of questions: "Which actors/institutions are responsible for monitoring and/or remedying this type of situation and making recommendations for action? Do adequate mechanisms, institutions and procedures exist to address the situation described through a human rights approach, and if not, how might these challenges be met?"[84] The human rights approach questions were almost identical to the public health set but integrated reference to a common activity in human rights advocacy: monitoring. The final set of questions was designed to bring the experts together, as suggested by the title, "Talking across Fields." Consequently, both expert groups were to consider ways the other group held expertise. Public health experts were to consider the questions, "How can *enforcing human rights* improve the quality and effectiveness of a public health intervention. Where might there be differences in goals or approach?" Human rights experts were to consider the questions, "How can effective *public health interventions* lead to greater respect for women's human rights? Where might there be differences in goals or approaches?"[85] This case, like the others, presented extreme circumstances but at least included many complicated realities of life (housing, immigrant status, reproductive health). Given the phrasing of the questions to the separate groups, we might assume that human rights experts were to monitor problems whereas public health experts were to intervene in problems. At the time, public health anthropologist Paul Farmer had published best-selling texts about health as a human right. Thus, the fact that the funder presented these two groups of experts as so different points to the context at the time: focusing on the intersection of approaches remained novel.

As another example of how differently some experts thought about these issues, we can look to funders' discussions of the viability of a human rights frame, which influenced grassroots programs. If funders could not shift their approach, many grant-dependent organizations would have one less incentive to do so.

The Ford Foundation commissioned a study of other philanthropic funders' perspectives on human rights. As a funder of domestic human rights activities such as developing SisterSong, Ford had a stake in expansion of these activities. The interviewees included over thirty current and former program officers, presidents, and executive directors of foundations, including the Ms. Foundation for Women and the Rockefeller Foundation. The title of the summary report, *A Revolution of the Mind: Funding Human Rights in the United States*, came from a quotation from HIV activist Carmen Barroso when she was at the MacArthur Foundation: "Human rights is a revolution of the mind with application in the real world." The report tried to retain an optimistic tone but was candid that expanding the "revolution" would be an uphill battle.

The largest challenge identified was the perception of human rights as foreign. Thomas wrote of

the profound separation that has arisen in the United States over the past fifty years between international and domestic rights activism or between human and civil rights work. Both consciously and not, many of the donors interviewed for this report held the view that the term "international" was somehow exclusive of the United States or that human rights was about abuse happening "elsewhere"; that is qualitatively different from the civil rights abuse occurring here. The prolonged estrangement between civil and human rights work has also left many with the impression that human rights is a "white, elite thing" about privileged Americans traveling abroad, while civil rights is a "more insular" field that has all but abandoned its internationalist past.[86]

The meeting contained explicit discussion about US exceptionalism, with people situated on either extreme, from pessimism to optimism, about challenging the exceptionalism. Thomas believed that "most fall somewhere in the middle: deeply concerned about the ramification of continued U.S. exceptionalism with respect to human rights and other issues like arms control and the environment, but uncertain if the benefits of challenging it outweigh the risks."[87]

Unsurprisingly, the report described human rights activists' movement presence in beleaguered terms: "peopled mostly by refugees from mainstream civil and human rights work." Refugees leave a country to save their lives, so using the language of "refugees" suggests that these activists had escaped other movements. By mentioning the "mainstream" of human rights activism, the report distinguished between types of human rights, thereby acknowledging that there was some level of support for certain forms of human rights, namely, political and civil, but not for others. Of course, it is arguable that there was actual consistent support for civil rights in the form advocated for by the early US civil rights movement—equality for African Americans. Yet, civil rights were a more familiar form of rights than social, economic, and cultural, which the report goes on to state activists desire to see. However, the report's merging—or conflation—of civil and human rights is important because this was an ostensibly knowledgeable author crafting a narrative in the form of a report that was undoubtedly to be read by funders and meeting attendees.[88] Thus, this conflation could lead to further confusion about the consequences of not investing in developing a grassroots human rights movement. The emphasis on the "indivisible" approach to human rights would continue to appear in different documents. The report was saying that people could not be selective when it came to advocating for human rights. Rather, all rights worked together.

A few of the donors opposed engaging the human rights frame, while almost half (fifteen) of the donors were identified as "interested (but undecided) in supporting human rights work in the United States."[89] One of these donors asked, "It is intellectually, philosophically and morally correct to look at U.S. issues in human rights terms, but is it the best way to work?"[90] A primary concern was backlash from the US government and foundation boards. For the "actively interested" donors (twelve), the positive aspect of a human rights frame was, among others, its basis in values, its emphasis on "indivisibility of rights" as "an approach that encompasses civil, political, economic, social and cultural rights," which found "resonance with 'grassroots groups,' with 'people and particularly women of color' and with 'young people.'"[91] At the end of the report, donors contended that they needed *other* bigger donors to take the lead. Donors placed the responsibility for funding US human rights activities in someone else's hands and checkbook.

A few years later, at a state-specific summit in Illinois, funders were again asked to reflect on the power they held to foment a human rights movement. The Illinois report again identified a key problem with human rights advocacy in the United States—the government would not shift its practices if its people do not demand that it do so. Thus, "Participants agreed that in the U.S. we often use human rights as a tool to abuse and punish other governments, but try to insure that we're not held accountable to those same standards at home. The United States will never be a more responsible partner in supporting international human rights conventions if Americans are not familiar with human rights and the protections and hope human rights offer."[92] The report also showed the possible influence of academic work: Larry Cox of the Ford Foundation recommended historian Carol Anderson's book *Eyes off the Prize* to attendees.[93] These conversations were important, but we can also imagine that if these rooms of philanthropic funders had moved forward in supporting human rights, it could have changed the funding landscape through which organizations navigated and would have certainly opened possibilities for advocacy.

Rights are contested constantly. Reproductive rights in particular face resistance from governments unwilling to give people higher expectations for healthcare, a fact recognized by agencies such as the World Bank that have a questionable history of interest in women's reproduction: "Given extreme financial and capacity constraints, the concept of rights may actually scare people away from opening doors they cannot control."[94] Yet, in a society with a comparatively high level of privilege, a generally nonchalant attitude towards rights poses a continued challenge to feminists advocating human rights. While this attitude is not only a challenge in the United States,[95] the consequences in the United States are partly the result of other movements committing to a constitutional framework that at its core emphasizes individuality. Despite these challenges, women of color activists forged ahead. So, once again, the question arises: why choose a human rights frame?

The women's movement's emphasis on gender equality under the law was insufficient. Equality assumed that men were the standard, but women of color argued that men of their communities also faced racism, just as they did. Racial equality, however, was also not enough to address the consequences of simultaneous racial and gender inequality that influenced the reproductive options of women of color (and poorer White women). Further, underlying economic inequality was not recognizable in either of these scenarios. Through a human rights frame, however, experiences such as forced sterilization, discussed in earlier chapters, could be understood as a violation of the "inherent dignity" of humans, which the first sentences of the UDHR have identified as in need of protection. Achievement of civil rights alone would not stop the systematic violations that these women of color and other marginalized members of society faced, but some opined that achievement of human rights could.

Part of the challenge was that there were several processes happening at once—collective development at the level of SisterSong and the intradynamics of the organizations themselves—so the development was happening as the collective was also looking to the future and to expansion. Yet, as I demonstrate in the remaining chapters, the initial hope expressed by some movement leaders about the possibilities for using human rights to achieve a range of reproductive rights was not universally shared, and its success far from a foregone conclusion. Rather, there was misunderstanding about human rights and ambivalence about their role in the future of the reproductive justice movement. That is where the origin story of SisterSong had an additional role to play besides merely documenting the collective's start: holding onto a narrative of *all* the key elements of the start, including a global connection. The March for Women's Lives provided a useful national forum for educating audiences and amplifying that narrative.

5

Marching toward Human Rights or Reproductive Justice?

The April 2004 March for Women's Lives was one of the largest single marches in US history up to that point, with over one million participants. Sociologists of the women's movement noted that the march showed that "the American women's movement remains capable of highly visible, large-scale, newsworthy collective actions."[1] How did the march come to be? In summer 2003, a coalition of four well-established national women's organizations—Feminist Majority Foundation, NARAL Pro-Choice America, National Organization for Women, and Planned Parenthood Federation of America—announced the march, then named the Save Women's Lives March for Freedom of Choice. Months later, the coalition changed the name to the March for Women's Lives. The new name indicated a framing shift, which represented a new organizing strategy that emphasized increasing the diversity of the march participants. The 2004 march differed from prior national women's marches because of its emphasis on diversity, social justice, and social issues beyond traditional "women's issues."

NOW had organized many national marches, including the April 1989 March for Women's Lives, which occurred during the George H. W. Bush administration to "let the Court know what would happen if *Roe* were overturned."[2] NOW described the April 1992 March for Women's Lives as having "leadership and delegations from every *pro-choice* organization."[3] While these are not the only national marches NOW has organized, NOW referred to both as "record-breaking" in the amount of support garnered, as demonstrated by the estimated numbers of participants: 600,000 in 1989 and 750,000 in 1992.[4] NOW noted that both "these mass marches forced *the issue of abortion rights* into the forefront of political debate."[5] The framing of these marches relied on a reproductive rights frame that emphasized protection of abortion and "choice" as the central goal of these demonstrations.

Previous accounts of NOW marches highlight that participation by women of color was startlingly low. In the 1986 march, approximately two thousand women of color marched.[6] In reflecting on the 1992 march, a newspaper from the National Black Women's Health Project estimated that only about one thousand people of color participated, despite their increased activism in the movement. The article described repeated attempts to meet with NOW's leadership (e.g., Eleanor Smeal) to include women of color in the planning. On a special conference call to discuss these concerns, Smeal left the call before the women could confront her with their complaints. While the agenda of speakers eventually included more women of color, the initial exclusion of these women increased frustration to the point that some women of color refused to attend that march. Many who did attend wore green armbands in visual protest against their initial exclusion from the agenda.

In a Management Circle meeting before the 2004 march, the irony of the position of women of color in the funding structure was noted: mainstream organizations were sometimes told by philanthropic funders that they needed to include women of color, yet, when women of color asked funders for grants for their own projects, funders challenged their ability to use the money. Consequently, some of SisterSong's leadership requests were quite blunt: "Stop giving mainstream organizations $ to do our work (Work in our communities)—because many of the projects they do are conferences, booklets, or other things that don't make a dent in the problems in our communities." Clearly, they did not feel mainstream organizations knew how to address the needs of women of color. Conferences and booklets, which can passively offer information, were grouped together. SisterSong had just held a large conference, so it was not that conferences, per se, could not be useful. Rather, Sister-Song critiqued the way mainstream organizations developed activities *for* women of color rather than *with* women of color. The 2004 women's march showed another forum in which mainstream women's organizations started with the "for-not-with" approach.

The 2004 march organizers initially framed the event as a response to an "attack" on reproductive choice, specifically abortion, by Republicans, including President George W. Bush. The external threat derived from his possible reelection. Organizers perceived the march as an opportunity to energize people through grassroots organizing around abortion rights that would defeat Bush come November 2004. The simultaneous threat *and* opportunity led to an unprecedented coalition by mainstream groups that sometimes competed on the national stage.

This initial diagnostic framing relied heavily on the language of reproductive choice and emphasized threats to abortion access. In June 2003, the four organizations announced the upcoming march, which was at the time named "Save Women's Lives March for Freedom of Choice."[7] While more than abortion was on the agenda, rights and privacy were still central in the diagnostic and prognostic framing, which proposed the solution to the problems.

NOW's earliest article about the march in the fall 2003 *National NOW Times* begins by discussing how, with "abortion opponents dominating two branches of government, infiltrating the nation's courts, influencing state policy and threatening to topple the landmark *Roe v. Wade* decision, the right to safe, legal and accessible abortion and birth control is in grave danger," thus marking the need for the march.[8] Here, the march represented collaboration by four major women's organizations to move forward the "abortion rights" movement.[9] With continual references to "abortion" (eight times), *Roe v. Wade* (four times), and "choice" (two times), NOW primarily focused on the march as a step in defending the right to abortion as guaranteed through the courts. Yet, as discussed in prior chapters, some women of color had been criticizing the "choice" analysis that made abortion and *Roe v. Wade* the most central reproductive rights issue. At the time NOW's march had the support of some unlikely partners, such as the United Farm Workers,[10] which indicated that some diverse groups supported the march even when the cosponsors were using the traditional "choice" framing. The march eventually expanded its base due to the presence of SisterSong at pivotal planning stages.

An interviewee who worked for one of the mainstream cosponsors recalled those organizations' leaders' discussions. Some leaders of mainstream women's organizations thought they were helping smaller organizations by conducting the majority of the work up front and *then* asking for endorsements. SisterSong was partially created to provide a space for women of color to repair what they felt were the negative impacts mainstream groups had had on the organizing power of women of color (e.g., draining of economic and psychological resources). Thus, some members considered the mainstream groups initially cosponsoring the march as "tainted allies."[11] Some of the younger members who knew this history explained initial feelings about the 2004 march in a film produced by women of color about the march. Malika Redmond, a national march coordinator, explained, "We marched with you in '92, we marched with you in '89 and it's the same thing we've been hearing over and over again. And we're tired of it because we've been saying that the struggles for marginalized voices are more than just 'choice.'"[12] Unsurprisingly, these previous conflicts meant that women of color wanted to have more control of the process when another march was proposed.

The year 2003 was a big one for the collective as it was when SisterSong held its first public convening. In November 2003, hundreds of people gathered at Spelman College for SisterSong's first public national conference. The conference had an estimated four to six hundred attendees. In the draft conference program explaining SisterSong to attendees, there was a note that "SisterSong is committed to a human rights framework. This framework is based on the early recognition among women of color organizers that we have the right to control our own bodies simply because we are human, and as social justice activists we have the obligation to ensure that those rights be protected."[13] While similar phrasing appeared in mission statements up to that point, this wording differed by tasking activists with guaranteeing protection of rights.

At the Spelman meeting, the second objective after building a US network was "to bring together women of color organizations, policymakers, advocates and health care providers to promote a human rights based approach to Reproductive Health and Sexual Rights."[14] Such an approach would be achieved in part through the "interrogation of narrow, excluding language of Choice-only rhetoric that does not speak to the sociohistorical and present day realities of Women of Color."[15] This was followed by the claim that "we prefer the more inclusive language of human rights and reproductive rights."[16] This was a confusing claim since "choice" and "reproductive rights" were at that time often linked—a critique SisterSong founders made—and both were associated with the right to make the choice of whether to have an abortion. Still, the larger context in which choices were made was emphasized.

Human rights also appeared to be foregrounded, as the second plenary was to make connections on "The Intersection of Human Rights,

Race, and Gender: Reproductive Health and Sexual Rights." The plenary included both activists and academics, with experience both in the US and internationally:

Patricia McFadden, PhD ~ Smith College ~ Author, *Southern Africa in Transition: A Gendered Perspective,* on "Reproductive Rights and Body Integrity"

Leila Hessini ~ Senior Policy Advisor ~ Ipas, on "Bush's War on Women"

Surina Khan ~ Former Executive Director ~ International Gay and Lesbian Human Rights Commission, on "Sexual Rights and Opposition by the Homophobic Right"

Andrea Smith (Western Cherokee) ~ Cofounder ~ Incite! Women of Color Against Violence, on "Population Control and the Right"

Euna August, MPH ~ Executive Director ~ Institute for Women and Ethnic Studies, on "The Reproductive Bill of Rights for Women of Color: A Tool for Advocacy"

Andel Nicasio ~ Dominican Women's Development Center (Centro De Desarrollo De La Mujer Dominicana), on "Identity and Gender"

The expansiveness of the issues covered in a plenary that focused on human rights is important to note. Given the titles of their talks, key movement leaders were understanding the interplay between the political Right and the influence of federal policy on women's bodies. Of note is that IWES's "Bill of Rights," referred to in other documents, was a focus as well.

Besides the plenary, two sessions had human rights in their title, one of which focused on international settings (Access to Termination of Pregnancy Services in South Africa, Gender-Based Violence and Human Rights in South Africa; and Reframing Civil Rights; Human Rights and Spiritual Rights to Advance the Reproductive Rights of Women of Color). Five other sessions included "human rights" in the description or paper titles. They ranged from how to use hip hop music in human rights education to how to understand the implications of C.R.A.C.K, the privately funded program that offered drug-addicted women money to get permanently sterilized, which, the presenter argued, "blatantly violates the constitutional rights and human rights of the marginalized men and women it has coerced into giving up their reproductive freedom."[17]

Despite the many other issues on the collective's literal agenda, connecting with activists from outside the United States also remained important. One set of notes offers an example of international exchange of ideas: "The Dignity and Justice U.S. Solidarity Tour of the Movimiento Independentista Nacional Hostosiano visited in March, as a Women's History Month event. Two of its leaders conducted a lunchtime presentation entitled 'Human Rights & Self-Determination for Puerto Rico: Women Led Struggles.'" Here was another example of drawing on a program that would construct international human rights discourse as relevant for the domestic political sphere. The Puerto Rican activists shared the history of the Puerto Rico independence campaign, including the status of that effort within the United Nations, with SisterSong staff and community members. The Latin American and Caribbean Community Center and Project South also sponsored the event. It is important to notice that the presenters talked about struggles with the UN. At times when SisterSong framed the organizing for human rights in the United States as a fight against powerholders who would not accept the UN and UDHR, they did not focus on the challenges groups face regularly *within* the UN structure. Sidestepping discussing these challenges makes sense, as it was substantial work to familiarize reproduction activists with the basics of the UN, so it was important to focus on its benefits. Still, leaders were aware that the UN could be a site of struggle even if the US government eventually embraced the UDHR.

At a February 2004 SisterSong Management Circle meeting held before the national women's march, explicit discussion of human rights and the role it should play in SisterSong's future appeared. One person implored, "The human rights aspect that SisterSong uses is extremely important and makes us different from other groups—acknowledging that we have multi-dimensional realities that have to be taken into account. *It is absolutely our strength, our uniqueness and should never be compromised. We hold a vision which may not be embraced immediately, but one that will catch on (as it already is) and gain momentum. No true movement or breakthrough concept was immediately embraced and free of controversy and lack of understanding.*"[18] This statement about human rights in SisterSong indicates that leaders understood human rights as a more comprehensive way to understand people's whole lives. The remark also demonstrates self-awareness on the part of SisterSong leaders that what they were doing was unusual: a "breakthrough concept" is by definition innovative. Despite the challenge promoting a new idea posed, Rodriguez insisted that it must "never" be compromised. By the time Rodriguez made this observation, SisterSong was seven years into promoting reproductive justice as connected to a human rights framework. That key leaders were still having conversations about the role of human rights points to the continued challenge of engaging with human rights discourse.

In the final part of the meeting, the participants divided into smaller groups to brainstorm the collective's five-year vision. One group's list included the idea that "SisterSong will nurture the health and well being of communities of color, raining down love, money." Again, attention to health as a broader concept served as a continuation of prior movement work such as that of the Black nationalists who focused on community health, as Alondra Nelson traces in her work on the Black Panther Party's efforts to connect "body and soul," as well as that of activists in the feminist health movement, who, in the words of historian Jennifer Nelson, longed for "more than medicine."[19] The image of "raining down love, money" further illustrates how SisterSong aimed to be more than a social movement organization or collection of them—it aimed to reconceptualize. Together, women of different racial and ethnic backgrounds could develop a form of health that benefitted the whole through commitment to both emotion and pragmatism. The summary list placed one set of ideas all on the same level, including the idea of human rights: "Happier Place/Long Term Hope/Self-Help/rituals /Holistic Approach to the work we do—human rights framework, intersection of issues/culture/analysis/strategy." These snippets encompassed ideas for both a strategy and a particular future. Thus, attention to human rights was conceptualized as both a process and a goal.

Making the Frame Shift Visible

Prior to SisterSong's November 2003 conference, it held a public conference call for women of color to discuss possibilities for endorsement. NOW had already announced the April 2004 march, so at this fall conference, representatives from each of the cosponsoring organizations asked SisterSong to endorse the march. Ross reflected on the endorsement request: "I thought it was particularly telling that of the four organizations . . . they didn't even all have women of color to send to represent them at our conference. . . . I have worked with you all 20, 25 years ago over this same question. You don't even have women of color in senior management?"[20] Indeed, NOW appeared to have the same problems that had generated earlier critiques of its limited racial diversity.

Eboni Barley, who became a march coordinator with NARAL, re-membered, "So in the beginning when we were not included in the planning process I was not only annoyed but I felt betrayed. . . . The SisterSong network really pushed for that envelope to be opened and we sort of opened Pandora's box with this March for Women's Lives."[21] After a conference plenary session at which attendees discussed the pro-posal, SisterSong agreed to endorse the march. Ross noted that younger women, who were more optimistic, were instrumental in making this decision.

SisterSong's endorsement of the 2004 women's march included stipu-lations. The first stipulation was to change the name of the march to broaden the emphasis beyond "freedom of choice," which, reproductive justice advocates pointed out, was often synonymous with the choice to have an abortion. A major part of SisterSong supporters' experiences was that their choices to have children were represented as irresponsible and pathological, as seen in debates around welfare reform and other policy discussions. Underlying the name dispute was the reality of dif-fering reproductive experiences, what should be done to improve the reality of those experiences, and how this reality should be presented. Of the names Ross proposed—"March for Women's Human Rights" and "March for Women's Lives"—the latter was chosen. While the new name ended up the same as that of a previous march, a sense of progress persisted because the name change would require significant financial investment.

The name change was part of a package of requested changes, some of which are described below. A new organizing campaign, New Voices for Reproductive Justice, was created to bring in women of color and other groups that had not been traditionally visible in advocacy for re-productive issues: its efforts and frame shift were visible. New Voices organized delegations from different cities to attend the march. A brochure inviting people to join New Voices explained, "With new constituents and issues at the table, future reproductive justice activism will seek to build a human rights–based movement that is truly universal and includes the needs of all women in the United States and abroad."[22] The hope that reproductive justice organizing would foment a commitment to human rights was clear—and that this could have global consequences was clearly also a goal. Further, including "new voices" would diversify the march at all levels: participants, leadership, publicity, and ideology. The brochure outlined the many "new voices" that would be present at the march: "New Voices includes not only the many unseen organizations and advocates of color who have historically fought for reproductive justice in communities of color, but dozens of organizations who are not widely perceived as being associated with the reproductive rights movement. Such advocates come from the anti-poverty and anti-racist movements, as well as those who work on HIV/AIDS, environmental justice, immigrants' rights, violence against women, and criminal justice issues."

A month after SisterSong's endorsement, NOW announced the change via the first e-mail to the march update listserv. The e-mail, which NOW duplicated verbatim in the winter 2003/2004 issue of *National NOW Times*, noted that the original name was too cumbersome, suggesting that the change was primarily for practical reason. However, the notice did incorporate some of SisterSong's language. More importantly, this e-mail is the first public document from NOW that used the phrase "reproductive justice."[23] Already, the framing was changing. The e-mail then describes the broader aim of achieving reproductive justice: "This March is about demanding political and social justice for women and girls regardless of their race, economic, religious, ethnic or cultural circumstances. This March is for young and older women, straight women and lesbians, sons and fathers, able and disabled, rich and poor to stand side by side in a show of unity and determination to 'never go back' and in fact, move forward with full equality and reproductive justice for all. The excitement is building!"[24] The announcement explicitly acknowledged the diversity in the category of "women" by referencing race, class, ability status, and sexuality while also including men in the effort. Further, the solution to the "attack" was urging the Supreme Court to protect *Roe v. Wade* and working toward "full equality and reproductive justice for all." The new name represented an underlying move from a traditional reproductive frame focused on choice to a broader reproductive justice frame.

Increasing Diversity—and Tensions—within the March Coalition

An article in the *National NOW Times* explicitly focused on the role of women of color in the march and emphasized diversity. The author noted that "fighters of all ethnicities, classes, ages, and sexualities" would be needed to stop President Bush, who was further identified as "violating human rights indiscriminately."[25] This language indicates that NOW was trying to link the problems involved in protecting reproductive choice to those involved in protecting human rights. Previous marches had not done this, but SisterSong explicitly incorporated these ideas into its materials.

Even after organizations have agreed to work in coalition together, they continually renegotiate the terms of their collaboration. Other conditions besides the name change included space on the planning committee (Ross agreed to become a march codirector), so that women of color were guaranteed to be included in the decision making. Ross hired Malika Redmond, a young African American woman who worked with Ross at the National Center for Human Rights Education, as a national march organizer. Redmond's responsibilities included coordinating women of color and other marginalized groups through activities such as identifying potential delegation leaders throughout the country. This was no small feat. La' Tasha Mayes, an African American Pittsburgh-area activist, discussed how she was skeptical about organizing a delegation when Redmond first contacted her. La' Tasha became more interested when Redmond explained that there was a specific effort to bring in "new voices," which Mayes saw as "so cool [and] so necessary."[26]

SisterSong leaders were wary of investing a large amount of resources when they felt that, historically, the smaller organizations gave up more to be involved with coalitions due to their limited staffing and resources.[27] So they wanted steering committee spots to be provided to some of the collective's organizations without the requisite $250,000 each of the other four organizations had provided as major cosponsors.[28] Thus, National Black Women's Health Imperative, National Asian Pacific Women's Forum (NAPAWF), the National Latina Institute for Reproductive Health, and SisterSong were eventually members of the steering committee. Problems continued to emerge even after the organizers changed the march name and more women of color were involved in the coalition. Jamie, a SisterSong member who was interning with NAPAWF when the march occurred, remembers her experience:

> I got to sit in on those meetings that were . . . extremely tense. You know, sitting there essentially with the old guard . . . you know sixty, seventy, eighty years old, White women who had been in the movement and felt that they had . . . defined the movement and that the movement was all about "choice" and all about abortion. And, um, this woman of color contingent being represented by various, you know, Latinas, African Americans, multiracial, Asians, API, and then just down the list of people that were like, "This is not our issue."[29]

Jamie described complex tensions that arose around both age and race, which other women also identified as creating tensions. An organizer for NOW, reflecting on her interactions in the field, felt that "many of the feminist[s], especially the older feminist[s] seem to take offense . . . that it was insulting to tell them that 'choice' was not inclusive of many women of color, low-income, and gay and lesbian communities."[30] Earlier feminists had defined abortion and its legal protection as the appropriate focus for the feminist movement's energy, hence the resistance to changing the frame as represented in even a small name change.

Locally, not all organizations had received word of the march's new name. La' Tasha, who organized a New Voices contingent for the march and later founded New Voices Pittsburgh, recalled a disagreement about the publicity materials a local group wanted to distribute: "They had . . . the old name of the March on them [March for Freedom of Choice]. And I was like 'Un-uh, we need the new card that says March for Women's Lives.' And that was significant but they didn't even know! They didn't know 'cause 'freedom of choice' sounded perfect [to them]. Obviously, that doesn't resonate with women of color, and it hasn't and they ask the question 'Why don't women of color participate?' I'm like 'Well, obviously, it doesn't resonate with them or their experiences.'" This newer approach of reproductive justice clearly resonated with La' Tasha and other members of her march contingent. Further, involvement with organizing the delegation connected La' Tasha to SisterSong, through which she eventually began organizing SisterSong's Queer People of Color caucus and joined the Management Circle.

Even though some of NOW's promotional material for the march still used language consistent with a reproductive rights frame, NOW's newer promotion emphasized the diversity of the march. The listserv announcements highlighted the breadth of partners, emphasizing the support of "nearly 1,000 cosponsors, including the NAACP."[31] Endorsements by major organizations like the NAACP, which had previously avoided taking a stance on controversial issues such as reproduction, did not come by accident. In an interview two days before the march, Eleanor Smeal, then with the Feminist Majority Foundation, credited Ross and other women of color with increasing the support for the march. She claimed, "The civil rights movement will be there, students from colleges and high schools will be there, women of color will be there. The environmental movement is coming—the Sierra Club has endorsed the March for the first time. We have more celebrities than I've seen before. We just have much more depth in so many communities."[32] The increased "depth" that Smeal describes demonstrates the increased success of the frame pyramid, which led to higher resonance with the march's adjusted framing, improving organizing efforts with women of color.

Beyond the name change, the extension of the feminist framing of reproductive rights was visible in other ways. SisterSong produced five thousand placards that it distributed at the march. Two feet by three feet in size, with a deep purple background and yellow lettering, the signs conveyed a festive tone, like Mardi Gras décor. The front side of the sign read, "Reproductive Social Justice for All Women." Since that march, "reproductive social justice" has been shortened to "reproductive justice," but SisterSong staff at times still described RJ as the merging (or "marrying") of reproductive rights and social justice through the human rights framework (e.g., at Reproductive Justice 101 trainings I attended and on the website). The flip side of the sign read, "Women of Color Taking Steps," which could be interpreted as both the literal marching and the process of moving toward a new analysis and movement strategy through which to consider women's reproduction.

One interviewee recalled a dispute about the text of the signs. This flip-side text about "taking steps" had not been part of the design that women of color leaders approved for final printing. Some felt that the addition infantilized women of color. In a 2007 RJ 101 training, Ross noted that there were not enough signs for all the women who wanted them. Further, there had been reports of a physical altercation due to a disagreement about whether White allies should be allowed to hold the signs.[33] Pictures from the march, including those on the websites of organizations like SisterSong and NOW, show many women holding the signs.

A photo from that 2004 march showed various people holding a yellow banner with large block letters stating, "Women of color for reproductive justice." The sign holders included various people of different ages and races involved with SisterSong, including Malika Redmond, Luz Alvarez Martinez, Dázon Dixon Diallo, and Loretta Ross. One person held a placard that said, "human rights educators for reproductive rights," making a clear link between the issues of reproduction and human rights. Other configurations of women of color carried that same yellow banner, along with the purple/yellow signs. SisterSong continued to use the purple/yellow signs at events, and the website contained pictures of the signs until a website revision in 2018.

While the march was advertised using the Internet, this was largely a pre–social media era, and thus the organizing occurred primarily through direct conversations, phone calls, e-mail announcements, and posters. Through the invoking of an intersectional analysis that linked reproduction to social justice and human rights, SisterSong also attempted to engage in frame transformation. It sought to move constituents to interpret reproduction not just as a matter of an individual's ability to make a private decision but also as connected to the conditions of whole communities, which should be protected by universally recognized human rights.

After the March: Moving Forward and Backward

After the march, SisterSong continued to emphasize human rights discourse in its work whereas mainstream women's organizations were less consistent in its use, although "reproductive justice" was used. The first issue of *Collective Voices* published after the march featured member testimonials about experiences at the march and SisterSong's role in the march. Another piece gave a short history of the organization and highlighted how SisterSong's analysis differed from that of other organizations: "The human rights framework shows that most people are denied many human rights entitlements. It addresses the right to healthcare, adequate housing, childcare, education, and social services. *SisterSong's mission is to connect reproductive rights to human rights.*"[34] This is but one example of the continued discussion of human rights in the emerging reproductive justice movement.

Some movement participants felt that an attempt to engage with the human rights–based reproductive justice frame showed concrete steps toward changing mainstream organization (and therefore movement) practices. But others, like Loretta Ross, remained skeptical. In an interview I conducted with Ross two years after the march, she reflected,

> The sad part is, though, despite the success of the march, the four mainstream organizations that started all of this mess, I think they saw diversifying the organizing as a great way to mobilize for the march, but I don't think they saw it as a great way to transform the movement into the future. Because immediately after the march, they went back to business as usual. Which is, you know, something SisterSong could have predicted that they'd do. They figured [it] out but they didn't. And . . . they somewhat lost the potential for using the women's human rights framework as a way of building the new movement. But that's what SisterSong is doing.[35]

Indeed, I would argue that the mainstream organizations' failure to capitalize on the success of the march helped SisterSong in some ways.

Did NOW not "figure out" the possibilities of an adjusted frame? On the contrary, NOW, like other SMOs, did figure out that a change in language could benefit the organization. For example, at the time, NOW's "Abortion Rights/Reproductive Issues" page introduction stated, "NOW affirms that reproductive rights are issues of life and death for women, not mere matters of choice. NOW fully supports access to safe and legal abortion, to effective birth control and emergency contraception, to reproductive health services and education for all women. We oppose attempts to restrict these rights through legislation, regulation, or Constitutional amendment."[36] NOW's "Young Feminism" webpage duplicated the paragraph under the section "Advancing Reproductive Justice—*Because My Body Is My Own.*" While NOW argued that reproductive rights were not just about choices, the first two components that the list focused on are two issues that are traditionally associated with organizing around reproductive "choice": abortion and birth control. NOW's affirmation relied on a rights-based approach: women have the right to abortion; therefore that right should not be taken away. The page encouraged readers to donate to "support NOW's work on abortion rights," which emphasized the need to protect abortion over the range of issues it purported to support. The page contained links to "related issues" NOW was working on: "Contraception" and "The Supreme Court," focusing on birth control and how laws explicitly afford or deny women access to abortion. Thus, NOW literally linked reproductive justice to abortion rights. If NOW was attempting to make a deeper integration of reproductive justice into the debate on abortion, one way to make the integration clearer would have been to link this issue page to its other issue pages, such as "Economic Justice."

The "Abortion Rights/Reproductive Issues" page linked to another page: "We want reproductive justice now!" The language on this page subtly reinforced the idea that abortion was the central concern regarding women's reproduction. Visually, the site attempted to show that NOW did address the concerns of women of color, or at least that the organization appealed to a larger audience than White, middle-class women. However, the page's introduction about the need for women's decision making to be "free from government interference" did not address how, as discussed earlier, some forms of government intervention would be needed to achieve reproductive justice.

In fall 2006, the *National NOW Times* featured an article on the differences among reproductive-health, reproductive-rights, and reproductive-justice analyses of reproductive issues.[37] Even though the organization was aware of the difference among these analyses of reproduction, NOW had not implemented this awareness systematically. These webpages provide an example of how a mainstream organization uses the rhetoric of a human rights–based women of color organization but does not incorporate it into its deeper analysis, which is indicative of limited frame extension. This illuminates a perspective voiced at SisterSong events and by my interviewees: "reproductive justice" is not interchangeable with "reproductive choice" or "abortion rights." Rather, reproductive justice demands a comprehensive reformulation of an organization's analysis and organizing around reproductive issues.

A younger activist, Jamie, observed,

> I don't think reproductive justice was new back when the march happened, but I think people started to understand that there—there's a difference [between reproductive rights and reproductive justice], they're not synonymous and that you know this is gonna be a movement about women's health. . . . At the end of the day that there are many issues that have to be brought to the table and considered and . . . just because something is legal or, you know, accessible, doesn't mean it's necessarily affordable for people. I think all of that really started to resonate with . . . women of *any* color.[38]

Another interviewee, Malika, identified the new language as indicative of "a shift in consciousness" that "put the knowledge production that was coming from women of color on the front stage." With this analysis "on the front stage," SisterSong led women of color (and their allies) to influence the framing of a national protest initiated by mainstream women's organizations. This solidified the importance of SisterSong. Mainstream organizations benefitted from increased visibility due to increased supporters, increased legitimacy for the attempt to become more diverse, and a new language to appeal to a wider audience when desired.

Before the 2004 March for Women's Lives, NOW had consistently talked about abortion rights and a woman's choice to have an abortion. NOW intended to frame the 2004 march in the same way and, as this chapter demonstrates, would have continued to do so if SisterSong had not joined the planning and required changes in exchange for endorsements. Leaders from NOW acknowledged that SisterSong's broader framework of reproductive justice helped the march develop into the largest and most diverse march in its history. SisterSong's success at shifting the framing of the march is the proof of its tagline, "doing collectively what we cannot do individually." The story of SisterSong's role in the 2004 march was repeated at many SisterSong events and in publications reaching hundreds of women of color (and allies), producing a narrative of credit in which a social movement claims influence over the outcome of activity around a particular issue.[39] The story both demonstrates why an organization like SisterSong exists and provides evidence that a reproductive justice analysis can be deployed successfully on a national scale.

NOW and other mainstream organizations' limited engagement provides additional evidence of the concerns raised by SisterSong that mainstream organizations claim to represent all women but in practice do not address the full life experiences of women of color, including the violation of their human rights. Whether mainstream organizations will more fully integrate this analysis remains a point of discussion among activists today.

Funding RJ Activism on Their Terms

As the collective grew, concerns about capacity building remained under discussion just as they had been at the founding. At the July Chicago meeting for the core member organizations, the training focused on key aspects of capacity building: self-help, the human rights framework, and applying for foundation grants.[40] Malika explained why trainings she held felt important: "Because I think our, from a domestic perspective, because often times people only understand the language of human rights from an international projection. So 'those poor people over there, those hungry people over there,' or whatever. And those are human rights issues. But then when we sort of think about ways that, like, you know, having healthcare connected to jobs, you know, that being a human rights issue, homelessness being human rights. You know, so starting to think about what are some of the domestic issues and framing it in that way."[41] These efforts were not constrained to traditional social movement organizations, as she described a popular education model of meeting people where they were, whether that was schools, churches, or community meetings, "to talk more broadly about social justice issues in the U.S."[42] Malika explained the importance of going to different types of community spaces to conduct human rights education. Further, she suggested that it was her specific interest— her women's studies background—that led her to emphasize women's human rights. That there was a special person designated to consider those issues rather than a general mandate to "infuse" the curriculum points to how gender considerations have historically been peripheral in human rights advocacy and a decade after Beijing still had to be addressed intentionally.

With the success of the march at increasing SisterSong's visibility, women of color still had to keep their organizational doors open. Educating funders was a continual process that organizers approached from different angles. In a climate where organizations competed for funding, being understood was of paramount importance. However, organizers described lacking the networks of mainstream organizations—or the trust of the funders. So, they took matters into their own hands. In conjunction with SisterSong's October 2005 conference, the collective members held a briefing for funders. The first goal was to "discuss and understand the Reproductive Justice framework and its basis in human rights." The sixth and last goal was to "learn from our colleagues in allied organizations and the funding community about the benefits and challenges of supporting organizations and programs that apply a Reproductive Justice frame to further and protect women's human rights."[43] The briefing booklet contained one-page summaries of the issue at hand. While only two of the one-page pieces had "human rights" in the title—one by Loretta Ross and one by Magaly Marques—the concept of human rights appeared early in discussions of the foundation and the uniqueness of the reproductive justice movement.

In describing the "pro-choice" position, various frames were labeled inadequate, such as "Women's Right to Choose/Privacy" and "Woman Knows Best." The authors identified that a limitation of the strategies around these frames was their failure to ask *for* government support: "All of the frameworks, except Reproductive Justice, emphasize a negative role for the government, an obligation to not interfere with private life decision-making. In doing so, these frames do not spell out the affirmative obligations the government has to ensure the necessary social supports for our decisions, such as eliminating the Hyde Amendment so that federal funds will pay for abortions for low-income women and women whose health care is provided by the Indian Health Service."[44] As discussed earlier, the *Harris v. McRae* ruling that upheld Hyde made clear that "indigency" could be a barrier to accessing abortion but that the government had not created the barrier and therefore did not have an obligation to remove it. So, the only way the US government could be interpreted as being obligated to fund abortions was through a human rights lens that referred to international human rights documents.

Emphasizing the strength of an intersectional perspective regarding both approach and identities, SisterSong noted the importance of expanding action beyond abortion rights: "By shifting the definition of the problem to one of reproductive oppression rather than a singular focus on protecting the legal right to abortion, SisterSong is developing a more inclusive and catalytic vision of how to move forward in building a new movement for women's human rights."[45] Inclusion, rather than being the downfall, would enhance activism. Further, the proposed movement was one specifically for women's human rights.

As the overview explained reproductive justice, human rights was visible: "Reproductive Justice states that women's reproductive rights are human rights and is a positive approach that links sexuality, health, and human rights to social justice movements by placing abortion and reproductive health issues in the larger context of the well-being and health of women, families, communities and nations."[46] The reference to nations is important here because in the later list of "standards" of reproductive justice, "Connection of local to global" was the second item. According to the list, reproductive justice activism needed to be "based on [a] human rights framework."[47]

In her contribution, Ross covered the history of domestic and international conferences that gave rise to the term "reproductive justice," described the eight categories of human rights, and finished by saying,

> In summary, SisterSong has three core Reproductive Justice principles that emerge from the human rights framework: 1 Every woman has the human right to decide if and when she will have a baby and the conditions under which she will give birth. 2 Every woman has the human right to decide if she will not have a baby and her options for preventing or ending a pregnancy. 3 Every woman has the human right to parent the children she already has with the necessary social supports in safe environments and healthy communities, and without fear of violence from individuals or the government.[48]

Note that at SisterSong events and in SisterSong writing, these principles were consistently shortened to "the right to not have children, the right to have children, the right to parent our children." Thus, while human rights sat at the conceptual core of the principles, there was not always inclusion of the phrase "human rights."

The other contributor who foregrounded "human rights" explicitly in a presentation was Margaly Marques, the executive director of Pacific Institute for Women's Health, which operated in California and globally. Marques focused explicitly on international connections: "Reproductive Justice beyond Borders: Promoting Women's Human Rights on the Domestic and International Levels." She referred to the "economic South" and noted that one of the three items necessary to build a movement was "shifting the dialogue on reproductive health to an inclusive perspective or social justice and human rights, including diverse social movements and international voices in the debate."[49] Again, the attention to the global in more than a cursory way was important.

Ultimately, the SMO documents show interest in human rights, whereas the funders' reports were more tempered. However, funders were only one audience, and there were many people interested in Sister-Song who needed other ways to learn about human rights. As I discuss in the next chapter, publications and convenings played an increasing role in educating movement supporters.

6

Writing Rights and Responsibility

In early 2002, SisterSong shifted from being a smaller collective of sixteen organizations to a broader membership structure; with this change, other organizations could pay for membership or affiliate status and individuals could become members, too.[1] While growth expanded the SMO's connections and reach, it also reduced control over the diffusion of ideas and material. Thus, SisterSong had a newer set of audiences that needed education, which required the use of different approaches. People potentially interested in the idea of reproductive justice but not part of formal organizations that hosted trainings or who could not attend events would need exposure to the ideas in other ways. Thus, the *Collective Voices* (*CV*) newspaper served as an important venue both for broadcasting a common message and for showing how women in other places experienced reproductive issues. Analysis of organizational publications shows how SisterSong used this format to do more than inform readers about interesting events. Rather, it was a forum through which to teach readers how to interpret the world and varying experiences through a human rights frame.

In this section, I focus on what I see as key to SisterSong's revolutionary domestication process: engagement in a framing approach I term "radical reaffirmation." It involves several discursive moves: first, making the human rights concept familiar (familiarity); second, legitimating the choice to pursue human rights through a broader narrative of the right to human rights (legitimation); and third, linking radicalness to identity (reclamation). Numerous examples of this approach abound in the newspaper, *CV*, and at events.

The Right to Know Your Rights

The newspaper offered another source of educating people about the relationship between human rights and reproductive justice. It had a circulation of eighteen thousand at its peak, although the distribution timeline was irregular. The text was like a typical newspaper, black and white, but each issue contained a different color theme such as purple text for the title of the newspaper, the titles of the key articles, and some pull quotes. Newsletter distributions that coincided with a specific conference, such as the Let's Talk About Sex! Conference, contained full color images throughout and were twice as many pages as a standard issue. The additional pages contained advertisements for upcoming events (e.g., the US Social Forum) or notes congratulating SisterSong on its accomplishments. Members received a physical copy of the newspaper in the mail, and extras were distributed at conferences and other events. SisterSong leadership invested in the newspaper, using it as a key source of information for and about the emerging reproductive justice movement.

In various pieces, SisterSong promoted the idea that human rights served as the basis of reproductive justice. One piece showed keen awareness of the lack of human rights consciousness in the United States, as demonstrated by its outlining of the process and consequences of human rights education: "The United States must be held accountable when violating international law at home or abroad. This can be done more effectively *when U.S. human rights activists become human rights educators to help people learn more about their rights.* Therefore, SisterSong advocates using the Reproductive Justice framework, a human rights–based approach that marries reproductive rights to social justice."[2] In this view, human rights education is necessary so people can better understand their rights and become better advocates for protecting human rights.

SisterSong core staff were aware that the inconsistent understanding of human rights meant lower likelihood of member organizations being able to educate their individual members. Here Heidi Williamson, who directed SisterSong's fledgling public policy efforts, explained,

> HW: Those of us who are inside the organization know that human rights is a part of the framework, but we've gotta do better at making sure that we are better advocates for human rights and what that really means for people of color in the U.S. because that is something that I miss. And that's something that a lotta people, even though they don't miss it, because they don't understand it, they kinda pull it out of the overarching definition of reproductive justice. And that's a lotta times where we lose people.

ZL: Lose people in talking with them or like in—

HW: In the explanation, we lose them in their ability to understand it, how they talk to other people about it. Like they just get lost. They don't understand it, they don't like it, it doesn't make sense. And because it's something that we don't talk about enough as just citizens in this country, like even if people get it, they still don't necessarily have the tools to talk about it to other people. And so that's how you really sorta change people's hearts and minds is to like empower them with the rule, with enough information to be able to talk about this and let the word, the definition spread by word of mouth.[3]

Heidi's response points to the complexity of education around human rights. People within the coalition needed to be trained to talk about human rights or lack of understanding would lead to skipping that part of reproductive justice discussions.

A *Collective Voices* article entitled "Reproductive Rights Are Human Rights" is an exemplary piece.[4] The piece weaves together history of the UN and treaties, US reproductive activism, and excerpts from UN documents. The UN documents are applied to reproductive concerns in the United States and then "translated" into plain language.

The piece re-presents language that probably appears "foreign" to readers and converts it into terms that are more familiar. From the outset, the piece notes people's lack of familiarity with the concept of human rights: "Reproductive rights activists in the United States underutilize the global human rights framework. This is largely because many are unfamiliar with the Universal Declaration of Human Rights (UDHR) and international treaties that protect women's reproductive rights. Reproductive justice advocates should become familiar with the human rights obligations of the U.S. government."[5] Lack of familiarity is identified as a key problem, which highlights the consequences of restrictive domestication.

Most of the piece follows the format of taking the text of a UDHR article, explaining it briefly in plain language, and then offering many contemporary examples. This section contains many examples of radical reaffirmation: "Self Determination Article 12: No one shall be subjected to arbitrary interference with his privacy, family, home or correspondence, nor to attacks upon his honor and reputation. Everyone has the right to the protection of the law against such interference or attacks.

Article 12 reinforces the concept of self determination. Government regulations and laws that prohibit a woman from accessing reproductive health care and sexuality education, whether in the form of anti-abortion legislation, welfare reform, or other restrictions arbitrarily violate a woman's right to privacy and interferes with her family."[6] The UDHR language is formal (e.g., "arbitrary interference") and could appear irrelevant to US audiences (e.g., attacks on honor). So SisterSong engages in translation to connect the ideas for the reader. The specific familiar examples brought in from the United States include sexuality education and anti-abortion legislation, presumably topics with which these readers would be familiar.

The article emphasizes that the UN documents under discussion are important because they provide a basis upon which to claim rights that go beyond civil rights: "Women have *the right to challenge disabling conditions* like poverty, environmental pollution, government policies, and corporate *practices that violate their human rights. This holistic approach* also recognizes the need to oppose race- and class-based *population control strategies*, and other human rights violations."[7] Human rights was identified as a "holistic" concept. Of note in this excerpt is that reproductive concerns were not identified as specifically *women's* human rights, but rather as general human rights.

Overall, taken together, this piece identifies the importance of the universality of human rights. The perceived ability of human rights efforts to address the *multiple* sources of a problem (e.g., racism and classism) is emphasized, offering an intersectional analysis. Further, the analysis integrated historical concerns about population control, which subtly identified the human rights project as being *complementary* to community-based efforts rather than opposed to them. This is significant because a common critique of human rights discourse is that Western superpowers invoke "human rights" not to advance justice but to advance democratic governments amenable to neoliberalism and thereby dominate other countries economically and militarily.[8] So here was a casting of human rights as useful in the pursuit of justice.

Another part of the piece referenced other countries, implying that SisterSong was just one site of human rights advocacy that was happening globally. Specifically, in a call to action, the piece notes, "Since the United States has not ratified either of these treaties [CEDAW or

GLOBAL VOICES

REPRODUCTIVE RIGHTS ARE HUMAN RIGHTS

Reproductive rights activists in the United States underutilize the global human rights framework. This is largely because many are unfamiliar with the Universal Declaration of Human Rights (UDHR) and international treaties that protect women's reproductive rights. Reproductive justice advocates should become familiar with the human rights obligations of the U.S. government.

Eight Categories of Human Rights:
Civil, Political, Economic, Social, Cultural, Environmental, Developmental and Sexual.

Reproductive Health as a Basic Human Right
Women have a basic human right to control their own fertility and have self-determination over their own bodies. Through a human rights lens, these rights go far beyond a limited focus on abortion to include the right to have and not to have children, basic health care, and treatments for reproductive tract infections, sexually transmitted diseases, and infertility. Women have the right to challenge disabling conditions like poverty, environmental pollution, government policies, and corporate practices that violate their human rights. This holistic approach also recognizes the need to oppose race- and class-based population control strategies, and other human rights violations. With this in mind, an honest assessment of international treaties and agreements affecting the lives of women is essential in creating an effective response to the current assault on reproductive rights and sexuality education.

The Universal Declaration of Human Rights (UDHR)
On December 10, 1948, the General Assembly of the United Nations adopted and proclaimed the Universal Declaration of Human Rights (UDHR), which was signed by the United States. The UDHR guarantees the human rights of all people and encompasses a broad spectrum of economic, social, cultural, political and civil rights. Articles 3, 4, 12, and 25 are important because they touch on major reproductive rights concerns of all women, particularly women of color. Despite the unfortunately sexist language used in 1948, women's reproductive rights are protected in the following articles:

The Right to Life, Liberty and Security of Person
Article 3: Everyone has the right to life, liberty and security of person.
Article 3 is perhaps the most comprehensive. Security of a woman's person cannot be guaranteed if a woman is not free, empowered, and enabled to make her own decisions about her reproductive health and sexual rights. This holistic approach considers not only the immediate aspects of reproductive health and rights, such as sterilization, abortion, contraception, sexually transmitted diseases, and reproductive tract infections, but also surrounding issues such as family and community violence, substance abuse, HIV and AIDS, health issues in prison, welfare reform, homophobia, access to quality education, and links with women internationally.

No One Shall be Held in Slavery or Servitude
Article 4: No one shall be held in slavery or servitude; slavery and the slave trade shall be prohibited in all their forms.
Article 4 speaks directly to decisions about abortion and contraception. Reproductive

rights activists have always defined forced pregnancies as a form of slavery and servitude in which parties other than the woman concerned decide the outcome of a pregnancy, forcing the woman to become a human vessel for a fetus. Involuntarily subordinating one human being to another human being's need is one of the essential definitions of slavery. While our society would never force a man to donate an organ to a child, we believe that it is acceptable to force a woman to give herself over to protection of a fetus. It is not only discriminatory, but it violates the fundamental human right to be free of involuntary slavery.

Self Determination
Article 12: No one shall be subjected to arbitrary interference with his privacy, family, home or correspondence, nor to attacks upon his honor and reputation. Everyone has the right to the protection of the law against such interference or attacks.
Article 12 reinforces the concept of self-determination. Government regulations and laws that prohibit a woman from accessing reproductive health care and sexuality education, whether in the form of anti-abortion legislation, welfare reform, or other restrictions arbitrarily violate a woman's right to privacy and interferes with her family.

The Right to an Adequate Standard of Living
Article 25: (1) Everyone has the right to a standard of living adequate for the health and well-being of himself and of his family, including food, clothing, housing and medical care and necessary social services, and the right to security in the event of unemployment, sickness, disability, widowhood, old age or other lack of livelihood in circumstances beyond his control. (2) Motherhood and childhood are entitled to special care and assistance. All children, whether born in or out of wedlock, shall enjoy the same social protection.
Article 25 explicitly states the enabling conditions and supports a woman needs to exercise her reproductive options in the most optimal conditions possible. A woman must have her basic human needs met, including access to health care and sexuality education, in order for her human rights to be protected. The article is inherently anti-essentialist: we all have the same human rights but we each need different things to protect them. It specifies that women and children are entitled to special care and assistance.

Treaty Ratification = Federal Law
However, the UDHR is not binding law; it is an agreement or recognition that nation states interpret however they see fit. Because of this, member states in the United Nations spent years turning promises of the UDHR into treaties that are legally binding upon the signatory countries. The following treaties are of particular interest to the reproductive rights and sexuality education struggle in the United States, both of which the U.S. government has ratified. When a treaty is ratified, it's the same as Congress passing a federal law. They are the Genocide Treaty and the Race Treaty.

Genocide Treaty
Jewish lawyer Rafael Lemkin coined the term genocide in 1943 in response to the systematic murder of Jews, Roma and other victims the Nazi government during World War II. Recognizing that the world lacked international laws and standards that would prohibit a government's aggression against its own people, the United Nations developed the Convention on the Prevention and Punishment of the Crime of Genocide, which states in part:

photo by Yaminah Ahmad

16 www.sistersong.net

Figure 6.1. Excerpt from *Collective Voices* issue 1.3

CVAW], an important goal of the U.S. reproductive justice movement should be to pressure Congress to ratify these treaties, bringing the United States into compliance with *the rest of the industrialized world.*[9] This phrasing normalized the choice of human rights within an *international* context even though it may appear radical and anomalous in the

SISTERSONG WOMEN OF COLOR REPRODUCTIVE HEALTH COLLECTIVE

COLLECTIVE VOICES

SisterSong P.O. Box 311020 Atlanta GA 31131 www.SisterSong.net 404.344.9629 info@SisterSong.net

Ningún ser humano es ilegal
Immigration Reform, Human Rights and Reproductive Justice

Vol. 2 Issue 5

By Laura Jiménez, Deputy Coordinator, SisterSong
May 13, 2006

Ningún ser humano es ilegal, **no human being is illegal.** This is one of the declarations made by immigrant communities and their allies at the protests, rallies, and marches throughout the United States in the last two months. In response to the proposed immigration reform measures being debated in both Houses of Congress, millions of people have participated in these actions, voicing their opposition to increased militarization of the border, as well as the more stringent and repressive enforcement of current immigration laws and harsher penalties for breaking them.

Although this newest set of legislation targeting immigrants appears to have set off the events and activities of the last two months, it is really only the most recent in a long history of attacks against immigrant communities in the United States. These recent protests are also linked to the 500-year history of social justice activism by Latinos and other immigrants that are ignored by the mainstream media. The real catalyst for the people's outrage is the everyday tension and indignity of having to survive under what amounts to blatant (and legally sanctioned) human rights violations.

SisterSong's Reproductive Justice framework understands that women make their reproductive health decisions within the context of their family's and community's life and circumstances. This is a perfect example of how an issue, such as immigration reform, will not only affect immigrant women of color, but also their families and their whole communities.

If Congress passes any repressive legislation, then we can expect that women will experience this debate played out on their bodies and in their realities. As stated in ACRJ's Reproductive Justice Agenda: "During a war, a woman's body is treated synonymously as the land: as a battleground where women and resources are exploited, and as a site where victors establish dominance by reproducing themselves in the population through women's bodies, as well as reproducing their values, culture, religion, language, and traditions." [1]

Immigrant women already have less access to reproductive health services for various reasons, including cultural and linguistic barriers, lack of health care coverage, poverty or low formal educational levels (which have been associated with under-use of medical services).[ii] If legal barriers are also erected, there would be the systematic, institutionalized and deliberate denial of the humanity of the people who are affected. In addition, other barriers include lack of economic resources to access medical services, and legislation that has already been enacted, such as the 1996 Personal Responsibility and Work Opportunity Reconciliation Act, which prohibits the states from using federal funds to provide Medicaid coverage for immigrants who have resided in the country for less than five years.

All of the immigration reform legislation currently being

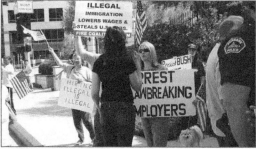

proposed in both Houses of Congress include tighter restrictions on services and benefits that could be accessed by immigrants. States including Arizona, Georgia and Virginia have already enacted such laws. It is critical to understand that, as this legislation is pending approval, the amount of public debate that is created by these proposals also trigger different types of behaviors from different groups of people:

• Undocumented immigrants who fear removal from the country stop trying to access services, causing medical conditions to go untreated, become emergency situations and create gaps in preventive strategies;

• Pregnant women do not access pre-natal services, causing poorer birth outcomes; and

• US citizens who work in institutions such as schools, hospitals, and banks among others, feel empowered to request immigration documents inappropriately, without guidelines and without legal authorization. This was the case immediately after California voters authorized the passage of Proposition 187 in 1994 (a law that denied social services, health care and public education to illegal immigrants and was subsequently struck down by the federal court).

In addition, we are concerned about the women who will continue to make risky attempts to enter the United States. According to the Committee of Indigenous Solidarity, "Rape has become so prevalent that many women take birth control pills or shots before setting out to ensure they won't get pregnant. Some consider rape 'the price you pay for crossing the border.'"[iii] More women than ever are attempting

such crossings with the full knowledge that rape and death are possible consequences. What will be their fate with the new beefed-up border security and the proposed 700-mile wall between the US-Mexico borders? What about the women who make the perilous journey in their last weeks of pregnancy with the desperate hope that their child will be born a US citizen? And what about the children and families that they leave behind who are depending on them for economic support?

These are all issues of extreme concern to the Reproductive Justice movement. SisterSong has supported and will continue to support the great number of immigrant communities and their allies that have come out in these recent events, and we support the movement for fair comprehensive immigration reform that recognizes and respects the human rights of all people. This recent public outcry has been a perfect example of an instance in which a unified Reproductive Justice movement has aligned itself with allies of other social justice and reproductive health movements to

Continued On Next Page >>

• US Social Forum pg. 10
• Mad At Birth Control pg. 9
• Latinas and HIV/AIDS pg. 15
• Women and Muslim Laws pg. 18

Figure 6.2. Excerpt from *Collective Voices* issue 2.6

domestic one. This legitimated the right to human rights—the implication is that if other people who live in the "rest of the industrialized world" can access these rights, people in the United States should be able to as well. Further, it allows for suggesting that the mechanism for change is the typical government structures.

The cover story of a 2006 issue that focused on the massive immigrant protests of that year provides another example of radical reaffirmation. The title proclaims, "Ningún ser humano es illegal: Immigration Reform, Human Rights, and Reproductive Justice." The article spans one and one-third pages, but features quite a few photos of protests. The first and largest photo is of a group of protesters waving US flags of various sizes, with homemade signs: "Hiring Illegals Is Illegal," "Illegal Immigration Lowers Wages and Steals U.S. Jobs," and "Arrest Lawbreaking Employers." Two of the people holding signs appear to be White women. In the corner of the photo, a uniformed police officer is visible, facing away from the protesters. The officer's shoulder patch displays "Burbank Police," indicating that this image is from Burbank, California, a state presumed to be progressive. A sliver of the officer's helmet is visible and a holstered gun is visible at the officer's waist. This all suggests police preparing for violence.

The article, penned by Laura Jiménez, SisterSong's deputy coordinator, begins, "*Ningún ser humano es illegal*, no human being is illegal. This is one of the declarations made by immigrant communities and their allies at the protests, rallies, and marches throughout the United States in the last two months."[10] The piece starts with a declaration that humans are not illegal. This claim tackles a common debate regarding immigration while also revealing a limit of humanism. In this case, the advocates challenged the conflation of a person having legal citizenship, which grants rights within a specific country, and a person's right to exist and flourish anywhere. The article continues, "This recent public outcry has been a perfect example of an instance in which a unified Reproductive Justice movement has aligned itself with allies of other social justice and reproductive health movements to declare, '*Citizenship, reproductive health, and the benefits that accompany it are not privileges; they are human rights!*'"[11] Discussing both privileges and human rights is also an important linguistic turn on the author's part because it clarifies for the reader that these are important distinctions. This statement serves two purposes. It educates readers and provides them a counterargument should they face a situation like the one displayed in the accompanying photograph.

Regarding the radical reaffirmation process, we see the different aspects of it. As far as step 1 is concerned, the concept of human rights being made familiar appears in a few ways. One is the simple connecting and claiming of immigrants as humans. As for step 2, the legitimation comes in the idea that human beings are in and of themselves "legal" just because they exist. Thus, humans have the right to human rights. As for step 3, there is an emphasis on movement identity—a collective identity as the reproductive justice movement, meaning that one allies with other movements and supports their efforts—in this case, gaining rights for immigrants.

Lest the reader think that only SisterSong staff wrote articles from this approach, it is important to note that guest pieces in the newspapers also provide evidence of the human rights approach. These guest pieces were written by members of organizations connected to Sister-Song in some way, such as being member organizations (again, keep in mind that organizations as well as individuals could become members of SisterSong). The same newspaper includes an invited contribution from Justice Now (JNow), a prison abolition organization that focuses its work on women in prison. The article has many functions: it addresses the specific issue of education on the experiences of incarcerated women, then contextualizes their experience. The piece explicitly identifies the organization's approach: "Similar to SisterSong, Justice Now uses the *international* human rights framework because it more fully encompasses the rights and responsibilities necessary for full Reproductive Justice."[12] JNow placed its work in a movement context by comparing itself to SisterSong and identified its work as having an *international* interest as well. However, there is the implication that the framework is not complete on its own, as indicated by the statement that the human rights framework "more fully" moves toward reproductive justice. The reference to "rights and responsibilities" offers nuance.

Later, the author explains point by point how a human rights frame could be applied to the situation of incarcerated women:

> First, Because women inside most often speak of their desire to have and maintain a family, we start with the right to family. The right to family is recognized in several treaties, in particular, Article 23 of the International Covenant on Political and Civil Rights (ICCPR) ratified by the United States in 1992. Article 23 states, "the family is the natural and fundamental group unit of society and is entitled to protection by society and the

state." General Comment 19, expanding on this right, stated "the right to found a family implies, in principle, the possibility to procreate and live together." In addition, the UN Convention on the Elimination of All Forms of Discrimination against Women (CEDAW), which the U.S. government has not ratified, protects the right of women to "decide freely the number and spacing of their children and to have the access to the information, education, and means to enable them to exercise these rights" in Article 16(1)(e).[13]

The radical reaffirmation process is visible through the steps of making human rights familiar by explaining which articles apply to the specific condition of incarcerated women, legitimating the choice of human rights by alluding to how the US government is an outlier in that it had not ratified CEDAW.

The author later explains how many women's experiences in prison could be interpreted as being in violation of human rights principles. This includes the right to healthcare, as the author notes the nuance in language: "This right to healthcare states that all persons are entitled 'to the enjoyment of the highest attainable standard of physical and mental health.' Article 12, ICESCR. Although it does not include the right to be healthy, the right does encompass the right 'to control one's health and body, including sexual and reproductive freedom, and the right to be free from interference, such as the right to be free from torture, nonconsensual medical treatment and experimentation.' ICE-SCR, General Comment 14."[14] While the analysis is subtle, the author is pointing out that although there is not a right to a particular outcome ("healthy"), there is a right to particular conditions, namely, control over one's own body. Thus, the article linked imprisonment to women lacking the right to control their bodies, which then leads to particular (reproductive) health problems that can have major consequences, including infertility.

While the piece concludes by emphasizing that the issue to address within the domestic context is the use of prison for punishment, the article notes that these circumstances are violations as viewed within the human rights framework. The author reflects on the position of movement actors: "Limitations on ratification and when the U.S. government fails to ratify human rights treaties (as it has failed to do so on most treaties) prevent individuals in the United States from securing these human rights through legal claims. Nonetheless, as activists we continue to use the human rights framework as our standard which should hold governments accountable."[15] The author offers the audience a primer on how to "read" common situations through a human rights framework while also exposing the reader to some movement strategy. There are some obvious ways in which human rights were presented as normal, for example, in advertisements for the collective's events. Part of the normalization of the human rights framework was the discussion of the *affirmative* role of government in human flourishing.

Leveraging the Ambiguity between Human Rights and Social Justice

Another key feature of the way SisterSong domesticated human rights was its leveraging of the productive ambiguity between human rights and social justice. At times, SisterSong used equivalence language, describing "social justice" and "human rights" as the same concept. I argue that this is in part due to restrictive domestication: with the audience ranging widely and having uneven exposure to human rights, there was a need to use different approaches to invite people to human rights. Use of the term "social justice" was one way to do that. At other times, the slippage between terms was due to leaders' own diverse relationships to human rights.

For example, at the 2004 March for Women's Lives, the signs that the women of color contingent printed said, "Reproductive Social Justice for All Women." This illustrated the close relationship between reproductive justice and social justice. In the first *Collective Voices* newspaper, which covered that 2004 march, the Latina Mini-Community's update noted, "Currently, we are working to adopt a Reproductive Health and Sexual Rights Agenda centered in a *broader health, social justice and human rights context*."[16] Here, the use of "and" suggests that these ideas are *not* all the same except in their connection to being "broader." Many issues of *CV* contained articles that used this phrasing.

The following year, the next issue of *CV* published a "Latina Principles of Community," authored by the National Latina Reproductive Health Policy and Justice Advocates. The brief "Principles of Unity and Equal Partnership," which called on advocates to endorse their agenda, included a goal: to "adopt a reproductive health and sexual rights agenda centered in a *broader health, social justice and human rights context.*"[17] This is clearly a repeating of the language used in the previous year's article. While this repetition could simply have been a matter of convenience, the *CV* issues were published a year apart, which offered enough time to choose a different phrasing; thus it appears that it was important to reemphasize the connection. In a front-page article in that same issue of *Collective Voices*, an interview with Loretta Ross offers a perfect example of this connecting of human rights and social justice. The first paragraph asks, "How do we build a movement for women of color for reproductive justice in the United States? Basically, *to ensure that the human rights of women of color* are protected, which includes reproductive rights. In this issue, we'll explain in detail exactly what is reproductive justice. *A shorthand definition of reproductive justice is reproductive rights married to social justice.* That is our ideal of reproductive justice."[18] Ross was—and remains—a masterful storyteller and writer. Her ability to pace a story, integrate surprise, and take the reader or listener down a path of discovery was obvious at every event I ever attended with her or when I met people who had heard her speak. She and others would repeat that reproductive justice was "reproductive rights married to social justice." As Ross was intentional in how she wrote and spoke, this specific way of presenting these ideas was probably not an accident.

The cover story "Reproductive Justice: Towards a Comprehensive Movement" details the history and efforts by various organizations within SisterSong. The author, Evenline Shen, who directed Asian Communities for Reproductive Justice (now Forward Together), noted,

Reproductive Justice is a positive approach that *links sexuality, health, and human rights to social justice movements by placing abortion and reproductive health issues in the larger context of the well-being and health of women, families and communities.* Reproductive Justice stresses both individuality and group rights. We all have the same human rights, but may need different things to achieve them based on our intersectional location in life—our race, class, gender, sexual orientation and immigration status. The ability of a woman to determine her reproductive destiny is directly tied to conditions in her community. The emphasis is on individuality without sacrificing collective or group identity. As with the human rights framework, it does not grant privileges to some at the expense of others.[19]

Here "human rights" appears as separate from "social justice," as evidenced by the need to link human rights *to* social justice.

A *CV* story on immigration protests highlights the range of issues around which immigrants were organizing: "SisterSong has supported and will continue to support the great numbers of immigrant communities and their allies that have come out in these recent events, and we support the movement for fair comprehensive immigration reform that recognizes and *respects the human rights of all people.* This recent public outcry has been a perfect example of an instance in which a unified Reproductive Justice movement has aligned itself with allies of *other social justice* and reproductive health movements."[20] Immigrant advocacy around human rights is an example of "other social justice," which positions both immigrant rights and RJ as social justice issues, not necessarily human rights movements.

Even in articles focused on the structural issues of movements, the ambiguous relationship between social justice and human rights is subtly referenced: "In response to the relative isolation of women of color *leadership in the reproductive rights and social justice movement,* and out of a real lived need to address growing disparities among women in mortality, morbidity, access to information and education, and economic and political power in the U.S. and the global context in general, independent and interdependent women of color led reproductive health and justice organizations have emerged."[21] In discussing the lack of women of color in key roles, the author identifies reproductive issues as "social justice" concerns.

This type of shifting of language was not simply a matter of SisterSong being in early stages. Later articles included this merging of language. The colorful double-sized issue of *Collective Voices* that Sister-Song published for the 2007 Let's Talk About Sex! conference featured a few articles and many advertisements/well wishes for the coalition's tenth anniversary. Again, we see the repetition of the common shorthand: "The advocacy agenda must include SisterSong's three core principles, which are: (1) the right to have a child; (2) the right not to have a child; and (3) the right to parent our children. These principles move us beyond identity and pleasure. They *marry social justice and human rights*."[22] Sometimes, even with more specific audiences, the relationship between the two ideas was not consistently elucidated. For example, the Funder's Briefing section, "The Problem Is Reproductive Oppression," explained, "From the perspective of SisterSong, *one of the key problems we collectively face is the isolation of abortion from other social justice issues that concern all communities.* Abortion isolated from *other social justice/human rights* issues neglects issues of economic justice, the environment, criminal justice, immigrants' rights, militarism, discrimination based on race and sexual orientation, and a host of other concerns directly affecting an individual woman's decision making process."[23] The text first identifies abortion as part of a range of "social justice issues." Then it clearly links social justice and human rights by pairing them. Here the "/" is visible to a reader as this is a written document, but it is an interesting choice. Using the slash mark rather than "and" implies that these ideas are so closely linked as to be inseparable even by a literal space. Thus, the reader is to understand that these ideas should not be considered as wholly separate entities.

Why does it matter if people think of "social justice" as related to domestic advocacy but "human rights" as related to international advocacy? Or, social justice as concrete but human rights as abstract? Or, the two concepts as the same? There are many reasons why these distinctions matter. Social justice is a less global vision than what radical movements of the 1960s and 1970s—or even anticolonial struggles of the 1940s—sought. Social justice is at times a parochial vision: if "social justice" is what is needed to achieve flourishing in the United States, if a movement were to achieve social justice, what would that mean for the rest of the world? Focusing on social justice can conceal US accountability to other nations. This allows people in the United States, even social justice advocates, to avoid considerations of how they benefit from US hegemony, which places them in a position of power relative to the majority of the world, even if they are not conscious of the power difference on a daily basis. Relatedly, the language of "justice" continues to connote a legal approach to solving social problems. Rights, justice, and legality are, for better or for worse, inextricably linked in the US public's minds.

This slippage in language also risks making human rights appear decidedly domestic, which people think of social justice as being. As with all movement strategies, there are advantages and disadvantages: there is familiarity, which can draw people in, but this can then create confusion when there is an effort to shift thinking: why try something that is new (human rights) when there is already a new concept (reproductive justice) bringing together areas that should be together? For many of the early movement leaders, the new concept, human rights, was the conduit for reproductive justice. But human rights as the larger goal means eventually getting to human rights, which is also why we see radical reaffirmation happening.

Still, some of the shorthand used is rhetorically useful but problematic. One conceptual problem with the idea of "marrying" is that it suggests bringing together *separate* entities since marriage brings together two separate people. Therefore, explanations like this position social justice and human rights as separate concepts. Practically, this makes sense in that it can help audiences quickly understand the concept of reproductive justice. That is, of course, a common practice in movements since they spend time crafting language to appeal to different audiences while also trying to maintain consistency. Further, there is the continued question of the reproductive justice movement being part of the human rights movement. If social justice and human rights are the same "umbrella," then everything is part of them, and that would not make human rights special. Yet, "human rights" is special in that it automatically connotes a global connection in a way that "social justice" has not. So, there is still a need to educate audiences about its specialness and implications.

In a *CV* piece titled simply "How to Talk about Reproductive Justice," Ross outlined her view of SisterSong's education process. The piece offers intramovement education and is about how to *do* intramovement education. Ross offers context on the necessity of education. She writes,

> *For many people, RJ is a totally new framework, and they concomitantly learn about human rights at the same time. For them, it is a life-transforming experience because of its power, depth and connectivity, especially to other social justice movements.* For others, RJ is a new phrase for a familiar worldview of intersectionality with which they have long operated. For both populations, techniques for talking about RJ may be helpful to overcoming resistance to a new way of thinking about reproductive health

and sexual rights issues, *especially in the United States that is obsessed with only talking about abortion isolated from other human rights issues.*[24]

From the outset, reproductive justice is discussed as a strategy for exposing people to human rights discourse. Ross paints a lofty vision of the power of learning about reproductive justice, saying that it facilitates a "life-transforming experience." However, it was clearly part of the goal of taking on reproductive justice. The first four parts of the approach Ross suggests are described by subheadings in her article: "Lead with Core Values"; "Discuss Obstacles to These Values"; "Use Self-help Techniques"; and "Offer the Human Rights Framework."[25] The list underscores how reproductive justice is process based. The values come first (parts 1 and 2), then the intramovement process of addressing personal problems (self-help). At a fundamental level, Ross was arguing for a need for basic education: "Since Reproductive Justice has its foundation in the human rights framework, it is necessary that people increase their familiarity with what is meant by the phrase 'human rights.'" This statement recognizes that people probably do not understand human rights, a consequence of restrictive domestication. Since it is key to reproductive justice, they need to better understand the ideas of human rights.

A *CV* article challenged the way some international human rights organizations were limited in their adoption of a human rights framework, with a focus on Amnesty International (AI). Amnesty International's early approach to human rights, which placed emphasis on political prisoners, is one with which people *might* be familiar if they have had any exposure to human rights discourse. In an article titled "Amnesty for Whom? Abortion as a Human Right: Amnesty International's Big Decision," Jiménez examines a possible vote by AI to consider supporting abortion rights. Since the vote was on supporting abortion in specific cases, Jiménez first challenged AI's logic, noting that "it does not address the underlying issue that all women must have the right to control their own bodies, whether as girls, when pregnant or when they are elders. Additionally, supporting abortion in these particular circumstances also sets up a dichotomy between those women who deserve and those who do not deserve this right."[26] This admonition offered the reader the opportunity to grasp the complexity of supporting abortion rights. The discussion expands beyond AI taking a limited view on abortion rights, to a larger set of arguments that occurred in movement spaces regarding abortion—namely, that arguing for the right to abortion based on exceptional circumstances was a slippery slope.

Then the piece went further in connecting a specific right—to abortion—to human rights. "In SisterSong's perspective, it is the responsibility of organizations such as Amnesty International and other human rights advocates to uphold the rights of all people to their own bodily integrity, and we believe that SisterSong, AI and others should not hesitate in putting this forward as a core part of our visions. . . . [A]dvocates for women also need to stand up and demand that women's rights be respected and protected. *Women's rights are human rights* and AI should understand these include sexual rights like abortion."[27] Making the point that women's rights are still part of human rights harkens back to the aforementioned struggle that began by advocates and academics bringing a gendered analysis into official human rights documents and advocacy. While perhaps seemingly obvious in retrospect, such a clarion call resulted from the challenge of having "women's issues" taken seriously. That AI's consideration was occurring forty years into its history indicates how politically challenging reproductive issues remained.

Yet, clearly Amnesty International was aware of a range of reproductive issues. In the same *CV* issue, a section titled "Reproductive Justice Round Up" highlighted three pieces of news. First, "Prisons Shackle Women Inmates in Labor" was an eleven-line paragraph.[28] The article cited AI statistics about states that shackle birthing inmates. Besides citing examples from specific states, the article ends with a quotation from Schulz, who is identified as the former executive director of AI. Including this article in the same *Collective Voices* issue as an article that criticized AI showed the complicated relationship with authoritative human rights organizations. On one hand, AI could be supportive on some avenues of reproductive justice such as the right to have children in humane conditions, while AI also had the potential to be unsupportive around other reproductive justice issues, such as bodily integrity. Thus, here the responsibility SisterSong demanded was for other SMOs, including a well-recognized human rights organization, to expand their understanding of "women's issues" and "human rights."

Global Connection and Concerns

Throughout SisterSong's narrative, the idea of a global awareness and a specific global responsibility appeared frequently. One obvious manifestation was discussion about the US government's responsibility to a global governance regime. However, another way SisterSong's idea of global responsibility emerged was in its claim to represent women globally and its sometimes stated goal of doing so. In other parts of the book, I give examples of the global connections SisterSong made with individual women and organizations outside the United States. For example, in preparation for the March for Women's Lives, there was a stated desire "to build a human rights–based movement that is truly universal and includes the needs of all women in the United States and abroad."[29]

Here I further discuss this narrative of SisterSong as embedded in—and sometimes leading—a global movement. At a basic level, SisterSong offered education about what was happening globally. It is important to remember that common news sources of today, like Twitter and Facebook, were not the widespread tools that they are today. Thus, SisterSong's newspaper offered a snapshot of issues relevant to the reproductive justice movement, the scope of which readers would not necessarily be presented with elsewhere. Thus, inclusion of discussion of reproductive issues outside the United States signaled that these *were* relevant to the RJ movement.

The first official newsprint version of *Collective Voices* included a multitude of articles: on conflict between women of color, SisterSong's next steps, and personal reflections on experiences such as the 2004 March for Women's Lives. One article was ostensibly reporting on the historic 2003 Spelman conference but went further in also describing the 2004 march.[30] The article starts off with a celebratory tone, claiming that the 2003 conference "was the largest gathering of women of color working on reproductive health issues in U.S. history" and detailing workshops, new projects that emerged (e.g., the Arab and Middle Eastern women's caucus), and the age range of speakers.[31] Then, the tone shifted to emphasize the gravity and potential impact of SisterSong's organizing:

> SisterSong believes that mobilizing thousands of women of color for the
> March for Women's Lives had a significant impact on the direction of

American society that is being deceived by a selected—not an elected—presidential administration. America is at a dangerous moment in history that is reminiscent of the 1930's in Germany when ordinary Germans did not understand the warning signs of their society. They were compelled into mindless hyper patriotism, whipped up into a fiercely aggressive war labeled as "defensive," misled by a government manipulated media that strictly limited access to alternative points of view, encouraged to express anti-Semitism, and most of all, urged to become debt-ridden consumers to prop up the German economy. The parallels to America today are frightening.[32]

The article provides a seamless—and perhaps on the surface hyperbolic—pairing: a women's march and fascism. By pointing to similarities in the political climate, the author wanted readers to understand that they were like the Germans, who could have made efforts to stop the rise of the Nazis. Lest the connection be too subtle, the next paragraph makes the connection between activism by US women of color and the global problem of creeping fascism: "SisterSong has committed to doing its best to help mobilize women of color in the United States so that *we take every peaceful action possible to stop this downward spiral of endless war and pitiless suffering worldwide.* The U.S. government is ceaseless in its attacks on women's human rights worldwide, most famously for its imposition of the Global Gag Rule restrictions that prevent women from having access to accurate sexual health information and that contribute to the 50,000 pregnancy-related, 3 million AIDS-related, and 75,000 unsafe abortion–related deaths worldwide each year."[33] The logic was simple: the US government had a global influence; therefore, SisterSong needed to have a global influence. So, participation in SisterSong activities was framed as contributing to *global* resistance against US policies that destroyed human rights globally. Far from parochial, the idea was to place SisterSong and its supporters in global context. This article offers another example of SisterSong creating a narrative that places its efforts within a historical trajectory that goes beyond that of the specific issue of reproduction or the work of existing SMOs.

The first issue of the *CV* newspaper most clearly foregrounded global concerns with a cover story titled "Globalizing Radical Agendas: How U.S. Policies Affect Women's Reproductive Rights around the World."

The author, Leila Hessini of Ipas Women's Health, sought to educate the reader on how changes in US politics had implications for women outside the United States, critiquing "the Bush Administration's euphemistic ideology known as 'pro-family.'"[34] Hessini argued, "The religious right and conservatives in the U.S. have joined forces to impose a radically conservative agenda on women domestically as well as around the world. This has resulted in countless policies and programs—often driven by politics instead of public health or human rights—that have curtailed women's health, rights, well-being and self-determination."[35] The article went on to discuss George W. Bush's political stances and policies while deconstructing a statement made by the US representatives at the World Congress of Families. This story illustrates how offering analysis of global politics was relevant to the collective. Further, it updated readers on the United States' role in global policy structure, reminding how domestic "local" concerns needed to be considered for their global impact.

The *CV* newspaper periodically included a section titled "Global Voices." Some of these stories were explicitly about organizing happening in other countries: "Women's Reproductive and Sexual Rights and the Offence of Zina in Muslim Laws in Nigeria,"[36] "Strategies of Resistance: Women Re-Interpreting the Meaning of Democracy in the Arab World,"[37] "Mobilizing Support for Community Health Workers in Trinidad."[38] In a later volume, an article of the same name ("Strategies of Resistance") included text that partially duplicated the prior article, but also covered different topics.[39] Another, "Beijing + 10: U.S. Proposed Amendment Defeated," explained the Beijing conference and abortion controversies and then went on to note the implications of SisterSong's participation in a women's health conference in India: "As one of the selected number of grassroots organizations and networks working in the global women's movement, SisterSong will help create a strategy to address growing militarization in countries, population policies and environmental issues plaguing women's health."[40] While there were only a handful of articles in the section formally titled "Global Voices," the news or ideas from outside the United States were included in each issue.

In another example of production of a narrative that placed the reproductive justice movement in connection with global activism, Ross contended that "women of color felt closest to the progressive wing of the women's movement that did articulate demands for abortion access who shared our class analysis, and even closer to the radical feminists who demanded an end to sterilization abuse who shared our critique of population control. Yet we lacked a framework that aligned reproductive rights with social justice in an intersectional way, bridging the multiple domestic and global movements to which we belonged. . . . We found the answer in the global women's health movement through the voices of women from the Global South."[41] In either case, there was reflection on the US government's policy and role in the international arena.

SisterSong primarily focused on domestic organizing. However, at various points there was some indication of engaging with women of color in other nations and a desire to represent all women of color globally. For example, a 2005 membership brochure proclaimed under "Our Mission" that "SisterSong is committed to being the global voice of women of color who are silenced by racism, sexism, and institutionalized oppression and abuse."[42] While on one hand the mission shows excitement about the possibilities of SisterSong, there is also a level of hubris in the thought that a US advocacy organization without any formal representation from internationally based advocates could serve as a "global voice." However, the claim to *represent* women of color globally potentially poses a different challenge if there were a more concerted effort to engage in those global spaces, such as conferences.

One way that SisterSong attempted to engage with women globally was through having people from other countries on conference plenaries to discuss how these issues operated in their country. Having international panelists may seem like a small gesture, but these speakers offered different perspectives both on content and on process. At events, these panelists would often discuss the process they had gone through to attend the conference, which for them required navigating the US visa system. Further, attending meant raising twice as much money as other attendees (or the conference organizers paying twice as much money to invite them). Thus, their stories explicitly and implicitly reinforced the necessity of attention to the intersections of nations in considerations of power structures. Another way of engaging women outside the United States was economic support. At one conference, SisterSong staff explained that they had intended to provide each registered participant a tote bag specially made for the conference by a group of South African women with whom SisterSong had a relationship through a member organization. However, there were no tote bags because a group of men had come into the women's workspace and destroyed the bags. The implication was that the men had acted out of jealousy of the women's economic venture. The story served to remind the audience that SisterSong had relationships with women outside the United States and financially supported women elsewhere (i.e., through commissioning tote bags). Further, it highlighted the importance of economic autonomy. Attending to intersectionality also meant developing an understanding of the way unmarked categories such as nation affected how specific forms of power, such as patriarchy, manifested differently across institutions.[43]

It would also make sense that SisterSong would need to embrace the human rights framework if it wanted to be relevant to individual women's movement organizations outside the United States, where women were already making claims in terms of human rights. The importance of the global would then be about more than connection—it would be about responsibility as US women of color. But continuing to hold that thread as a point of solidarity poses a challenge. As Falcón has written, US women of color were also challenged on their connection to US imperialism when they traveled to other countries, an uncomfortable position for some US women of color unaccustomed to viewing themselves as part of the reproduction of global inequality.[44] Notably, Falcón found that US women of color engaging in UN processes at meetings about racism, such as Durban, were taken to task for not understanding the extent of US imperialism and US foreign policies.[45] It is one thing to say that an organization is connected to an imagined global sisterhood, but it is another thing to experience that connection.

Human Rights as a Return to a Civil Rights Legacy

Another important tool to legitimize human rights was framing human rights advocacy as a return to the civil rights movement and the movement's "real" intention. Loretta Ross's explanation of the role of human rights in the development of CHRE exemplifies the approach of recasting human rights as civil rights:

And so I actually had a chance to ask one of my mentors, a Reverend C. T. Vivian, who was the board chair for the Center for Democratic Renewal where I'd been working, about the human rights framework, and he surprised me. . . . And he went on to say, "Martin meant to build a human rights movement." And he actually showed me copies of Dr. King's last Sunday sermon, where he called on us to build a human rights movement and then he was assassinated four days later. And so I was like, "Well, why hasn't nobody done this?" I mean, why, in 1995 nobody's done it. And then he says, "I don't know." And I said, "Well, certainly we can't fight for rights we don't know about."[46]

Ross's story, which was retold at various SisterSong convenings, provides a narrative of a different way to envision the civil rights movement while legitimating the reproductive justice movement. Radical challenges had long been part of an ancestral (racial) tradition, linking to other radical efforts.

In this narrative, a human rights perspective is presented as the next obvious step by Ross, who noted that a much-revered US civil rights movement leader *intended* to take this step. The narrative allows for a rhetorical turn in which the reproductive justice movement is both an extension of a past movement *and* the future of a movement. The juxtaposition of King's last sermon and his assassination suggests that the idea he was moving toward—human rights—was so radical that it had to be contained. Thus, SisterSong had the duty to continue this radical legacy.

Embodying Human Rights at the "Mother House"

In-person training activities also reinforced the idea that a human rights framework was integral to reproductive justice. Reproductive Justice 101 trainings lasted two to seven hours depending upon the forum (e.g., a shorter conference workshop versus a full training offered at the national office or requested by organizations). An e-mail advertisement for an October 2007 Atlanta workshop started with a reference to *Roe v Wade* and the "conservative shift of the nation," then pointed out how women of color are "disproportionally affected by cuts to Medicaid, dangerous contraceptives, welfare reform, immigration restrictions and more."[47] The linking of a range of issues besides abortion alluded to the potential scope of reproductive justice. After proclaiming, "We are ready for change!" the advertisement provided the answer to where that change would come from: "SisterSong is offering new vision for a winning movement: Reproductive Justice! Reproductive Justice calls for the complete physical, mental, spiritual, political, social, and economic well-being of women, girls, and individuals, based on the full achievement and protection of human rights." This was the fuller definition of reproductive justice that Asian Communities for Reproductive Justice had developed in its 2005 publication, "A New Vision." A photo from the 2004 March for Women's Lives showed a group marching behind the yellow banner that stated "Women of Color for Reproductive Justice." Also visible are the purple and gold signs stating "Women of Color Taking Steps." Even three years after the march, its iconography was being used to mobilize potential movement supporters.

I attended the full-day training at SisterSong's Mother House in southeastern Atlanta. The two-story green house had been the location of the National Black Women's Project and now housed SisterSong and SisterLove. It was set back at the end of a winding driveway, but remained visible from the street. As with other houses in the neighborhood, iron security bars covered the windows, and there was an iron security door. While the ironwork design had a floral pattern, the security bars and door subtly indicated that people were concerned about possible burglaries. Laura Jiménez, the deputy director, greeted me. The wood floors, high ceilings, and windows imbued the space with a light air. To my immediate left in the entry hallway hung a large, colorful quilt. I recognized the quilt from SisterSong's 2007 Let's Talk About Sex! conference. One of the cultural activities in which conference attendees could participate was to make a quilt square. After the meeting, Cara Page, national director of the Committee on Women, Population, and the Environment, did the physical work of stitching the squares together into the large quilt that now hung in SisterSong's office.[48] On the right side of the entryway sat a low bookshelf with newsletters from other organization, copies of SisterSong's newspaper, and fliers, including my own flyer for interviewee recruitment.

As I stood in the hallway, I asked Laura about my role in the workshop since I was there as a researcher. She laughed and said, "C'mon you know we are interactive," showing me to the room. When workshop participants entered the Mother House, we received a heavy blue folder and a staff person directed us to the main meeting room. The main meeting room was at the back of the house, so the large windows overlooked a back porch and parking lot. The room also held a library with built-in wooden bookshelves containing various books and newspapers. The group of about twenty people, who appeared to be almost all women of color, sat at round tables. I recognized people who had attended other SisterSong events and a couple of public figures I had interviewed months prior. One participant was Mia Mingus, who codirected Georgians for Choice along with Paris Hatcher, the two serving as the organization's youngest executive directors. In addition to her work on reproductive issues, Mingus regularly spoke on panels about her experience as a transracial Korean adoptee with a visible disability (she often used forearm crutches). I recognized Cara Page, who had spoken at both SisterSong's Let's Talk About Sex! conference in Chicago in May and the first US Social Forum in Atlanta in June.

As people waited, I perused the folder I had been handed upon entry. The glossy, light blue cover had the SisterSong logo and a collage of photos. Some of the photos appeared to be stock images, but I recognized others as conference photos. The folder had about ten items in it. The first was a small booklet with the title "Universal Declaration of Human Rights" with the logo designating it as from the NCHRE. The first paragraph explained the origins of the UDHR, which "established the moral standards for the indivisible and inalienable rights due to all humans."[49] The next paragraph put the United States in context: "However, the United States has not yet fully embraced the principles in the UDHR. Because Americans enjoy a variety of human rights every day, we tend to associate the human rights movement with the unrealized rights of political prisoners or ethnic minorities abroad. Instead, the UDHR prompts us to recognize that injustices occur inside our borders. When a family is homeless, when a school provides inadequate education, when people with disabilities are denied universal access to buildings, when a woman is beaten or raped, or when a hate crime is committed, these are human rights violations." The idea was to help the imagined US reader who held the booklet in his or her hand understand that human rights violations surrounded them. The bulk of the booklet was the actual text of the

UDHR's 30 Articles. The final page included a call to action to create a broader US human rights movement and NCHRE's contact information. The booklet's placement as the first item in the folder highlighted the clear connection SisterSong sought to make between itself and the concept of human rights. Other items in the folder included handouts of the PowerPoint slides for the day, a SisterSong Funder's Briefing report, pages from the press packet that outlined the history of SisterSong, a timeline titled "Evolution of the Concept of Reproductive Justice," and a donation envelope.

The morning began with Loretta Ross welcoming us and reviewing the day's agenda. We took a pretest with questions about our understanding of human rights and reproductive justice. In the next half hour, everyone introduced themselves. The slide prompted us to share our name, political work, organization/city/state, and what we wanted out of the training. Many participants identified themselves as staff or members of local or regional organizations. Some people described themselves as generally interested in the topic but not experts. One participant's introduction included the qualification that "I don't do political work." One young woman explained her interest in the training as based in her life story. More specifically, her mother, who sat next to her, had used drugs while pregnant. So, the young woman said she felt happy that she had been born "healthy," because something bad could have happened, such as being born "with a disability or something." No one commented on her characterizing disability as "bad." My introduction, as always, included that I was a researcher, which explained why I had traveled all the way from Michigan. A mix of seasoned activists and community members were all so eager to learn about reproductive justice in more depth that they were willing to spend a sunny fall Saturday indoors.

The workshop contained several sections with activities and breaks integrated into the main sections. In order, we would learn about SisterSong Core Reproductive Justice Principles; Origins of Reproductive Justice; Reproductive Oppression; Intersectionality and Human Rights; and Reproductive Justice—Strategies, Key Players, Constituents.

The reproductive oppression section introduced the idea of "self-help" as a process that could address human rights violations since it "[r]eveals stories of human rights violations—acts of humiliation and exclusion, [v]alidates a person's humanity and acknowledges the whole range of emotions that we experience and [u]ses self-disclosure to get in touch with painful moments to initiate a healing process."[50] SisterSong's form of self-help differed from the one promoted by popular press books or even in other spaces inspired by the women's movement.[51] Here, self-help was *explicitly* political and encouraged personal reflection in service of political change toward human rights.

When we got to the section of the workshop that was to focus on "Intersectionality and Human Rights," one slide was titled "8 categories of Human Rights." The section facilitator, Dázon Dixon Diallo, provided an overview of the history of human rights and referred to the Eastern Bloc countries. She also noted that some rights not originally recognized in the UDHR were added later, like environmental rights. The facilitator explained, "'It's your right to do' it put a different spin than 'It's the right thing to do.'" The facilitator reiterated, in laypersons' terms, the implication of human rights: people *already* had these rights rather than needing to persuade governments to give them these rights. We had a right to these rights. Based on the expressions on various participants' faces, this idea was an intriguing proposition. As Roberts reminds us in his interpretation of Arendt, there is a difference between making a claim to belong to a group that deserves rights and belonging to that group.[52] The facilitator proposed both our rights and our belonging.

On a practical level, the rights discussed existed in the UDHR, but governments still would have to create policies for people to be able to exercise these rights. That was not part of the early section of the training. Next, we moved to an interactive portion of that section. First, the facilitator had everyone stand up. Then, she read five statements:

1) I have lived in a neighborhood with unsafe toxic conditions
2) I have had problems accessing benefits because of my language, or other issues, such as same-sex relationship
3) I have not had access to health care because I didn't have insurance
4) I have had unprotected sex that risked transmission of disease
5) I have experienced violence in a relationship[53]

After reading the statements, the facilitator asked us to sit down if we could answer "yes" to *any* of the statements. Two people remained standing; according to their introductions, they identified as a queer Black man and a young Black woman. Someone asked, "So what does that mean?" Diallo replied, "We're coming for you." Her reply garnered some laughs although there was no explanation of what exactly she meant: SisterSong wanted to draw on those people's resources? Or, eventually the "we" of oppressive social institutions would enter their lives? Or something else?

Despite the ambiguity, the activity offered a moment of levity amidst what is often an emotionally intense experience for people—discussing oppression and privilege. All these statements addressed health, broadly defined. Upon further assessment, it is apparent that these statements focus different levels of intimacy, government responsibility, and individual responsibility. For example, while we could argue that these are individual choices at some level, there is a difference between having unprotected sex with a specific person and living in a given neighborhood, which could be largely based on where one's parents lived, where one's job was based, or simply what one can afford. People across the political spectrum can learn a different language, whereas there would be disagreement about people being able to learn a different sexual attraction. Still, the point of the exercise had been made through an auditory and visual technique: in any given space, most people faced a commonality in experiencing barriers to health, which was somehow a violation of their human rights.

Another activity we did that morning included identifying human rights violations. The facilitator went through different examples of rights, including sexual rights. We were about to read vignettes highlighting specific human rights and their violation, but first a woman at a back table asked a question. Specifically, she was curious about men's rights in intimate relationships: "So, that means he has a human right to have sex with me even if I don't want to?" The other participants' expressions ranged from curiosity to disbelief as they waited for the facilitator to answer. In some ways, the question was not an unusual one. Indeed, in many ways it represented a level of confusion and misunderstanding shared among participants in the reproductive justice movement. The facilitator explained that, no, one cannot violate someone else's rights to achieve one's own human rights.

However, as the workshop proceeded, the challenges of intramovement education about intersections of identity and experience rose to the surface. At lunchtime I sat outside on the deck with a few attendees, including Mia and Cara. Mia asked us whether, the next session, she should point out the problem with the comment about disability. No one had challenged the young woman's framing of disability as "bad." On one hand, the lack of intervention made sense as the training offered a space for people to tell their stories as they understood them. Yet, in the young woman's telling, she had posed disability as a negative health outcome, which denigrated the existence of at least one other participant. When the larger group reconvened for the afternoon activities, Mia raised her concern and there was brief discussion. However, it was clear that if Mia had not taken it upon herself, the comment would not have been addressed. Thus, I saw in action a point Mia, and some other interviewees, had raised in their interviews: inclusion of people with disabilities in reproductive justice activism was not at the forefront of people's minds. Accordingly, the workshop unintentionally highlighted a few tensions. Intersectionality that operates on an "inclusion" model of bringing oppressed groups into spaces is a limited mechanism for change as larger institutions structure our thinking about each other; thus more systemic change is necessary.[54] There was the ideal—learning about human rights across sectors, connecting people most affected by various oppressions and holding different privileges among themselves to create a stronger reproductive justice movement—which bumped up against the reality of people entering a movement with different levels of understanding of a range of issues, not just reproduction and human rights.

The RJ 101 training introduced people to the collective's origins, the scope of reproductive justice, and the idea that human rights are *in* our lives (or should be). An exercise offered in the advanced training (RJ 102) pushed on the complexity of understanding individuals' relationships to human rights. In "Reproductive Justice & Human Rights—Victimized Violators," participants were encouraged to engage in a multipart reflection:

1) Name a time when your human rights were violated
2) Name a time when you violated someone else's human rights
3) Name a time when your human rights were protected[55]

Of note here is that the exercise conceptualized human rights slightly differently from the way scholars emphasize human rights. Scholars often focus on how the state creates, protects, or hinders creation of the conditions under which human rights are respected. In this model, human rights violations can only occur when a government does not live up to its obligation. The first and last statements of the exercise echoed traditional, more obvious ways to understand human rights. But the middle statement explicitly asks participants to stretch beyond state-centric models to consider how their own actions could have violated someone else's human rights. In SisterSong's model, turning the analysis toward one's own actions facilitates understanding human rights as a relational practice between individuals.

These workshops offered single opportunities to learn about human rights. Also, it is important that movement leaders were mixed in with "average folks," so we would expect different levels of exposure to movement concepts. Other opportunities to learn were at the Let's Talk About Sex! conference in Miami, where one of the preconference half-day workshops was on human rights. There was not a follow-up to the workshop, but certain concepts were emphasized throughout trainings and through other fora such as newspapers.

True change occurs when people internalize different ways of thinking and align their action with those thoughts. Culture change does not occur only because the government legislates it or courts rule on it. The history of the US civil rights movement demonstrated this point: legislative approaches can have the unintended consequence of backlash.[56] Thus, by actively analyzing human rights in their own lives, participants were to come away understanding their relevance and that changing the US government's approach was not the only requirement for securing human rights. Transforming participants' understanding of their past experiences into new terms, providing them a framework to evaluate their relationships to other people, is part of the way to make human rights familiar. This shift matters since it also has the potential to empower members most directly, most immediately, by suggesting that they have the power to make human rights real. The power is not only in demanding that the government act but also in how people act in their own lives. Acting in one's own life was also about creating a human rights culture.

In sum, through this framing approach, SisterSong focused on culture shifts both within the reproductive movement sector and in connected movements. Building movement by increasing the size of the coalition and securing more funding was part of the initial aim, but so was attention to the process through which that would occur at both the individual and the movement level. Without attention to process, movement participants could unwittingly reproduce the underlying problem (violation of human rights). Culture shift is one of the hardest activities in which movements engage and can take years, if not decades. It is important, however, to shift the way people understand human rights as a worldview or set of guiding principles so that it is core/foundational. This is the case because keeping discussions at the surface can be useful for initial motivation, but persuading people on the basis of surface understanding of ideas means that they can be more easily persuaded in a different direction. So, the goal is to shift human rights to a deep place, of being so embedded as to make them a guiding principle of action for women of color. This sometime means making human rights appear simple and obvious to audiences. Human rights were sometimes presented as inevitable, logical, and obvious. At other times, human rights were presented as a more complex possibility. Talking about human rights as international contributed to the image of the organization as in the vanguard and pushing the envelope. In some ways that is what is happening. However, it was also the case that various human rights institutions had roots in the United States due to the early meetings about the UN occurring in San Francisco.

Further, some global voices had pointed and would undoubtedly continue to point to US imperialism as a source of the problems *other* women faced. Housed in the United States, having engaged with domestic social movement primarily, and still figuring out the best model for its own organizing efforts, SisterSong could not feasibly speak for all women of color. However, the desire to do so would of course mean that there would need to be a global consciousness and, ideally, a global action. Part of fomenting a culture shift of US activists would be understanding the domestic sphere as global, and vice versa.

It is one thing to identify a grievance as broadly a human rights violation, but SisterSong was offering a reading that could help members (or, in this case, any readers) understand murkier situations. Human rights framing was presented as simultaneously radical yet familiar and better than but not opposed to other popular framing options, including the civil rights frame. I propose that it was the very absence of human rights as an ideologically resonant claim in the United States that played a large role in SisterSong's revolutionary domestication. Leaders acknowledged that the United States was involved with UDHR creation, but presented human rights as a global phenomenon. Thus, taking on the mantle of human rights advocacy in the United States was joining with an array of other countries.

Radical reaffirmation allowed for suggesting the "radical/familiar" and "both/and" quality of movement identities and framings. Hence, this shift to human rights can be best understood through an intersectional analysis, a feminist approach to research and political practice that considers how people's experiences are constituted through multiple identities.[57] This allows for a "both/and" framing of human rights—and the problems it identifies as being relevant to (e.g., reproduction)—rather than the "either/or" framing common in other movement contexts.

Transforming participants' understanding of their past experiences in new terms, providing them a framework to evaluate their relationships to other people, was part of the way SisterSong understood success. Building movement by increasing the size of the coalition and securing more funding was part of the initial aim, but so was attention to the *process* through which that would occur at both the individual and the movement level. For some, human rights represented that process.

7

"They're All Intertwined"

Developing Human Rights Consciousness

This chapter focuses on interviewees whom I term "learners" because they understood themselves as being in the process of learning about human rights. For example, my study recruitment material referenced "human rights," and I began the interview with an overview of the broad topics about which I would ask. Yet, many interviewees struggled to find the words and the specificity to discuss human rights when I asked directly. In contrast, many interviewees referenced other subjects without my prompting, such as racial conflicts in the women's movement or how funders influenced the programming SMOs pursued, neither of which were topics in the interview protocol. I place other interviewees in two remaining categories of "skeptics" and "integrators," who were at either end of the spectrum. Both demonstrated an understanding of human rights, but had contrasting responses to that understanding: rejection versus embrace. At the end of the chapter, I discuss integrators, who intentionally integrated the human rights frame in their praxis.[1]

The Distance of Human Rights: Space and Race

Echoing what I observed at the RJ 101 workshop, many interviewees' responses point to the consequences of restrictive domestication, the US government containing the definition and scope of human rights. Notably, when reflecting on their understanding of human rights, many interviewees expressed initially not understanding human rights as a concept that appeared relevant to their lives. For example, in a number of interviews, when I asked what interviewees had meant when using the term "human rights," they began their answer by referring to examples outside the United States, and some even used the qualifier "international." The focus on the international arena speaks to the consequences of the US government's restrictive domestication—they first thought of human rights violations as existing elsewhere. With few opportunities to learn about human rights, for many in the United States, human rights can appear foreign, or at least irrelevant.

Taja, a Black woman who chaired SisterSong's public policy working group at the time of the interview, considered her previous exposure to human rights: "The human rights framework? No . . . so I hadn't really had too much exposure to much of anything. I knew about the UN and it wasn't really resonating with me as this huge bureaucratic process and entity. It wasn't really, wasn't a space that I felt connected to."[2] Taja explained how she had limited knowledge of the concept of human rights. In college, education focused on "problems" that felt like "railing against what's not working, what hasn't worked, and kinda the violence that's been committed, in a very liberal arts kinda way." The "liberal arts" approach, presumably with an emphasis on critical discussion, had felt abstract to her. What knowledge she did have at the time was associated with an international apparatus, the United Nations. Thus, she had not felt the relevance of the "bureaucratic process" the UN represented. Human rights, mediated by an image of a distant UN, was specifically *not* resonating with her experience. She contrasted that with "reproductive justice," which she felt provided solutions. This association among human rights, bureaucracy, and discussion of problems—without solutions—limited the appeal of human rights to her.

Perceiving human rights as "out there" presupposes that human rights differ from civil rights. Again, this is understandable since full human rights, unlike civil rights, remain outside of most US children's formal education. Even if people in the United States are unfamiliar with the specific details of the US Civil Rights Act, for example, most can still point to key leaders (e.g., Martin Luther King Jr.) and key moments (e.g., Rosa Parks refusing to give up her seat on a segregated bus) in the civil rights movement. Civil rights are emphasized in schools and in the media through designated days and months designed to highlight them, documentaries, and TV programs—all showing the process of people making civil rights claims through the US legal system. This is not to say that this level of knowledge is enough. At the 2017 *Los Angeles Times* book festival, Representative John Lewis's staff member Andrew Aydin referred to the "nine-word" problem of the US civil rights movement—specifically, that people's knowledge of the US civil rights movement is limited to nine words: "Martin Luther King" (Jr.), "Rosa Parks," and "I Have a Dream"—two visible figures and the title of one of King's speeches.[3] On one hand, reducing decades of struggle to nine words is probably discouraging for movement activists and academics. On the other hand, this is probably more information than people know about social movements that have not been integrated into the US school curriculum or had a key leader acknowledged with a national holiday.

The US government offers no equivalent socialization or acknowledgment of human rights: few people in the United States have opportunities to observe how the UN works or to learn about human rights in the terms internationally recognized outside the United States (i.e., a broader set of rights well beyond civil and political rights, including socioeconomic, cultural, and developmental rights). Programs like Model UN, in which young people role play as delegates and debate policy, are optional, with limited scope.[4] They are connected to local chapters of the UN Association, which are concentrated in politically liberal states, and various chapters are based on college campuses, where people are already privileged enough to pursue higher education. So, in the United States, formal opportunities for learning about human rights remain sporadic at best.

The perception of human rights as "academic" also made some interviewees characterize the pursuit of them as impractical. In an earlier chapter, Sonya, one Latina interviewee who helped found SisterSong, is quoted as saying that she thought the idea of human rights was new to many women founding the collective in the mid-1990s. Her response highlighted how human rights discourse can appear both inaccessible ("academic") and literally like a foreign language to learn. Since people discussing human rights appear to have advanced degrees and/or be elites working in international governmental organizations, human rights can appear out of reach or even irrelevant to people in the United States focused on grassroots work in communities removed (or even excluded) from these discussions.

For some interviewees, human rights initially felt unappealing because of their association with privileged people advocating on *behalf* of rather than *with* the marginalized people experiencing the violations. "Mehra," an Asian Pacific Islander interviewee, suggested that this trend influenced some people's understanding of human rights: "I feel like the jargon of human rights [belongs] in . . . kind of a corporate-y like White non-profit I guess. [laughing] But then the more I thought about it, I was like . . . somebody else has taken this term and made it kind of like sterile and kind of not . . . really political . . . when they do it. There's no justice about it. . . . So it just never really spoke to me in the same way."[5] For this interviewee, human rights appeared "out there" due to her associating such advocacy with both inauthenticity ("corporate") and racialization (for White people). Her linking whiteness with human rights points to how understandings of human rights are both embodied and political. Thus, while people of color might be most in need of protection of their human rights, the image of White people directing the helm of advocacy had deterred people like Mehra from being interested in them.

Other research has provided evidence that international human rights organizations are becoming more focused on professional expertise and engagement with the technicalities of human rights law, rather than grassroots empowerment.[6] The degree to which people thought of human rights organizing as the purview of elites correlated with their own reluctance to participate in broader human rights mobilization. Although some critics will claim that people do not need to have experience with legal structures regarding certain rights in order to have those rights, that perspective discounts the importance of experiential knowledge.

Epistemology of Human Rights: Learning the Language

This brings us to the various ways of learning about human rights. To be sure, many interviewees could not remember exactly when they first heard the phrase "human rights." However, they could describe key sites of learning. A couple of interviewees who were raised outside the United States or with family members in other countries recalled learning about human rights early in their lives. However, they were the exception.

Formal Education

One interviewee, Jaime, a biracial staff member in a genetics education organization, remembered the phrase "human rights" being mentioned in her early education, but its specific meaning had not been explained. She was, however, able to better understand human rights through legal training later in life. Jaime provided a detailed description of human rights and their implications. She learned about human rights as a law student in a specialized law course that was intensive enough to be termed an "academy":

> I didn't have the exposure. . . . I'd heard the term, and I was like, "yeah, that sounds really good." But, you know, I was never taught about human rights anywhere in my public education, upbringing, all the way through high school. Rarely heard it in college and had to physically seek it out in law school. And, you know, like I attended the human rights academy at my law school and that was my first immersion into it. But we don't, I think if it's talked about here it's so often talked about as atrocities that are happening out there, Darfur, um, you know, and not to take anything away from the tragedy and the genocide that's happening there, 'cause it is tragic and does need urgent attention. But there are all these other components. And if you, I mean part of the beauty of human rights is that you, your country's supposed to provide what it can provide at that time, so it recognizes that there are certain places that aren't financially able to sustain a universal healthcare system. But the U.S., I mean, how many times over could we have done it with all this funding that's going into the Iraq war?[7]

In her response, Jaime provided a detailed description of human rights and their implications. Additionally, she notes that human rights again seemed more "out there," as indicated by her using the exact phrase and then referencing Darfur. Further, she understood the ways in which government obligations to provide conditions for exercising human rights are weighed against having the resources to do so ("aren't financially stable"). Like Jamie, Amanda, a White woman, also had exposure to human rights in law school. She noted, "I was doing litigation for that clinic. So, I wouldn't say that was super RJ-related, although, you know, we did learn about the international human rights framework and sort of women's rights as human rights and reproductive rights as human rights. We covered those things in an academic sense." Both Amanda and Jaime had extensive exposure to human rights discourse through their legal training. However, this made them exceptions compared to other US interviewees.

Law school serves as one means of exposing a new audience to human rights, but legal codification is only one aspect of human rights. The formal (legal) aspect of human rights is most like the way civil rights are approached in the United States—via litigation. Yet human rights are norms, practices, and relationships that go beyond law on the books. In contrasting reproductive rights and reproductive justice movements, Amanda associated "rights" with lawyers. Yet, she noted, "[What] I like about the RJ framework and movement is that it's not a lawyer-centered movement. And it's, you know, like lawyers' skills are certainly welcome and needed but they're not the end all, be all." Having learned about human rights as a legal regime, Amanda associated human rights with the professionals who also dominated reproductive rights advocacy: lawyers.

Specialized legal education about one aspect of human rights does not automatically lead to understanding the multiple facets of human rights. Rather, it encourages people to view human rights as an extension of US legal practice, even though many are not currently viewed that way by courts and cannot be litigated for as such since they are not in the Constitution. While the Supreme Court has been inconsistent about considering international law in its proceeding, some argue that there has been a "recent departure from its tradition of doctrinal isolationism."[8] Still, legal human rights education represents a narrow opportunity for professional elites, and reinforces the idea that human rights are only useful to lawyers rather than the average person.

Learning about Human Rights within International Settings

In my interview with Tonya, a Black woman working at SPARK RJ while completing a doctorate in political science, I noticed that she referred to "human rights" frequently early in our interview. It was unusual for an interviewee to do so, so I asked her where she was first exposed to the idea of human rights. She identified the influence as coming from working with Afro-Latino activists: "Human rights, probably doing work, when I started doing work on Afro descendants in Latin America. Maybe six, seven years ago. Domestic human rights, five years ago. Which is very different because most people aren't grounded in the application of US-based human rights organizing, advocacy, or academic work." In her response, Tonya clearly articulated the idea that people in a range of US settings were not "grounded" in human rights. Still, she went on to explain why a human rights framework resonated: "But, so I would say human rights because, particularly in Latin America because of the way in which Afro descendants and other marginalized groups, workers, had to utilize international human rights fora as a way in which to vocalize the issues which are happening inside their countries because of the oppressive military dictatorships that most people were living under at the time during the '70s and '80s, and just, you know, finishing up in the '90s when, you know, democratization really took."

During the interview, Tonya named a few of the US–based organizations that she said "of course" had been founded by women, like the NCHRE, which Ross had directed. But this is all in the context in which, as she noted, US-based advocacy was not something with which people were "grounded." This lack of grounding is a consequence of the US government's restrictive domestication. Yet, as Tonya's answer highlights, there may be other reasons why some groups in some countries are more open to the human rights frame, such as experiencing military rule and needing to seek recognition through other mechanisms.

Correspondingly, "Lucie's" European upbringing familiarized her with the human rights framework. She worked at an international women's health organization and experiences human rights as a "basic" framework to interpret the world. However, the strength of her viewpoint was a rarity and stemmed from her relatively unusual exposure to human rights principles. She was the only interviewee who mentioned learning about human rights during her early formal education. She quickly recognized the difference between US and European education around human rights while attending a SisterSong training:

> And they [SisterSong staff] were going through the whole training and they spent a huge amount of time going over human rights and what they

are and they were specifically saying, "We appreciate that the majority of people haven't even heard of these things." . . . Not like I was fresh off the airplane but like "What? This is very different" [laughs]. That [human rights] was sort of the basic concept of social studies in high school for me and almost before. It was not an alien concept, the concept of human rights, as it was sort of presented in that [SisterSong] training as something new that we needed to be introduced to.[9]

Lucie's experience highlights some of the national differences in human rights education. She learned about human rights as "the basic concept" in the core curriculum from an early age in Europe. Further, she failed to realize the degree to which peers raised in the United States lacked such exposure until she attended a SisterSong workshop, much like the one I described in an earlier chapter. The workshop presenter's assumption that "human rights" were "alien" to attendees surprised this interviewee. Moreover, it is worth reiterating that even this training was not something that most Americans would experience, unlike lessons in school about civil rights.

Another interviewee, Maame-Mensima, an intern at SisterSong's office, noted being more familiar with "human rights" than "social justice." This was a rarity among interviewees, but she was another interviewee who had some international connections in her upbringing:

I guess because of my background—my mom's from Ghana—I've always been interested in international work. And with international politics, you see a lot more human rights work on the grassroots level. So, my exposure to human rights work has been a lot higher before I came to SisterSong. And at one time, and I'm not throwing it out the window, I've thought about doing like a master's or a PhD in human rights work, you know, international development. So human rights, as an example, has been a part of my intellectual upbringing or education for as long as I can remember.[10]

She was one of the few interviewees who had exposure to human rights earlier in life. Further, she identified her personal connection to an academic interest in international settings. Maame-Mensima, like Lucie, offers an important contrast to many of my interviewees. Both women grew up in environments where human rights were discussed regularly. As a result, they came into the reproductive justice movement perceiving human rights as relevant to their own lives. While this may be an obvious point, their experiences help illustrate the effects of restrictive domestication. Unlike the other interviewees, these two avoided those effects. Tonya, as an interviewee who eventually worked in spaces with international communities where human rights discussion was the norm, became comfortable with the language and ideas through repeated exposure.

Learning about Human Rights through Exposure in SisterSong

Many interviewees explicitly mentioned SisterSong as the site of their initial exposure to human rights, or their initial understanding, beyond a general awareness of the phrase. For example, the eight categories of human rights were referenced at different points in my study. There were opportunities for passive exposure, such as when visitors went to the website, which, for at least a year, contained an image explaining the eight categories of human rights.

However, there were more active ways of learning about human rights through SisterSong. For example, "Gina" worked for a women's organization that she felt facilitated her understanding of human rights due to her contact with SisterSong: "And it really wasn't until I started working here and networking amongst other organizations in SisterSong that I was able to make that connection in a concrete, tangible way."[11] Gina's comments point to the production of human rights consciousness as a collective process of educating and interpreting experiences *as* human rights issues. This collective process of developing human rights consciousness was not only for people with the least exposure to human rights.

Laura, a Latina SisterSong staff member, reflected on SisterSong's role in her own learning process: "Yeah, human rights was not ever my, it's not been my base of learning. Like that wasn't something I learned and that I'm learning, well, until I came to be a staff person at Sister-Song. And of course because I work with Loretta [Ross] and she knows human rights like back and forth, up and down, you know, in her sleep. So I'm starting to be able to articulate what human rights has to do with reproductive justice."[12] Beyond "starting to" articulate the relationship, Laura facilitated part of the RJ 101 training and wrote pieces for the *Collective Voices* newsletter that discussed the relationship between human rights and immigration issues.

Another staff person, Heidi, a Black woman, also noted the importance of SisterSong for deepening her understanding of the relationship between reproductive justice and human rights:

> I think the only thing that may have really shifted for me is sort of understanding more the human rights foundation of it. That was never really part of my understanding until I had to start doing the [SisterSong] trainings. And even now, I still think we aren't going far enough in talking about human rights and how much that legal document, like the Declaration of Human Rights, really sort of bolsters our work. And in part we don't because, you know, a number of our members and a number of the people we deal with are uncomfortable with that. They don't understand it, it's not a part of the conversation around like the rights of women and people inside the U.S. It's always about what rights and protections people outside the U.S. have as it relates to human rights.[13]

Here Heidi acknowledged that some SisterSong supporters and other organizations were not comfortable with the language of human rights. As she describes why, it becomes clear that she is pointing to the consequences of restrictive domestication: people understand human rights as relevant to "people outside the U.S." Heidi's comment also points to an unintended consequence that other staff members discussed: teaching other people about the explicit relationship between reproductive justice and human rights enriched her own understanding, thereby increasing her comfort with the human rights framework.

Mehra, a Middle Eastern woman working on the West Coast, elucidated the important role SisterSong played in providing a praxis of human rights. Mehra emphasized that SisterSong brought life to the idea of "human rights." She elaborated on her earlier point about previously viewing human rights as "corporate-y":

> Ok, so human rights I think I always saw as international and social justice I think I saw as like tangible ways that people are making a difference

about human rights. . . . I feel like the jargon of human rights is like very much like a kind of a corporate-y like White non-profit I guess [laughing]. But then the more I thought about it I was like, yeah, this really is. It is human rights, you know, like there's, *just because somebody else has taken this term and made it kind of like sterile and kind of not really, it's not really political I feel like when they do it.* There's no justice about it, it's just like, yeah, people shouldn't be hungry and people shouldn't live with violence and the state shouldn't be oppressive to them. But not like the, really like these are people and it's really important. So it just never really spoke to me in the same way. *Like I've always cared about them but I think human rights through SisterSong, it's much more compelling. I think it's just more personal.*[14]

The evolution of Mehra's view on human rights suggests that other interviewees could also positively conceptualize this framework. Specifically, she noted that after a SisterSong conference, human rights appeared more justice oriented to her, suggesting possibilities for reconfiguring human rights consciousness. Presumably, SisterSong, as a women of color organization, had provided an image of human rights advocacy that was different from a "corporate-y like White non-profit." SisterSong's approach could be seen as advocacy *with* a community in need rather than *for* a community. Interviewees' responses, such as Mehra's, emphasize the importance of organizational exposure and interaction around human rights to actively understand human rights as a framework for domestic issues. Ultimately, who is physically engaging in the human rights framing can play a pivotal role in interpretations about their relevance.

The Direction of Human Rights: Ground, Umbrella, and Thread

Below I discuss key ways in which interviewees articulated understandings of human rights and the implications for movements trying to organize using human rights. There were multiple approaches to human rights that I conceptualize as having different directional components: under, over, and through. Human rights as an overall concept was understood as simultaneously "under," providing a foundation for life; "over," providing protection from harsh elements of the outside world; and "through," providing a connecting link between ideas and people.

Some responses exhibited all these ideas at once. However, this is not indicative of misunderstanding or indecisiveness. Rather, it demonstrates the multifaceted capacity of the human rights framework. The human rights perspective is all of these things at once, which is both its promise and its peril.

Grounding Human Rights (Under)

Some interviewees described human rights as basic or foundational, which suggests that they are a place of stability. For example, Michelle, an Indigenous midwife working in the Southwest, acknowledged a lack of formal knowledge of the exact terms.

> I just don't see how it couldn't be human rights. And basically my reaction, and I've said this in SisterSong meetings before, is like this is a human-centered conversation, what we're having, reproductive justice. We're only talking about human justice, human reproductive justice and human rights and human justice. That's so far all we've discussed. And it's important, that's what we need to do, you know. But so I can understand why, of course, to me it's a no-brainer. Of course this is a human rights issue. And I just don't see how it couldn't be, you know. I really don't know what the international, I haven't like read the international definition of human rights, but I'm pretty darn sure that if I did, I would, that's, my reaction would be okay, of course, of course, you know.[15]

Although Michelle said she lacked formal knowledge of human rights, she communicated that she would "of course" support this framework. This statement indicates a trust in the concept by proxy—others have engaged with the ideas and found them worthy, so there is a "vouching" for the utility of the human rights lens. Further, her knowledge of human rights seemed sufficient for her to be asked to serve on SisterSong's Management Circle.

A different interviewee, a White college student, Ashley, encompassed what she thought were specific human rights:

> Human rights is *inherent* rights that all people have. You know, to live a happy, healthy, and sustainable existence, you know, and try to be in

harmony with other people and animals and the world. And so things like, you know, everybody has the right to healthcare, everybody has the right to food, everybody has the right to housing, everybody has the right to live in a place where they aren't affected by like conflict and warfare. And, you know, everybody has the right to choose who they have sex with and, you know, who they can love. And defining, human rights are just sort of *the bare essentials* of what make us people.[16]

Ashley's casual referencing and placement of a panoply of social goods shows how free-floating *and* encompassing people can believe human rights to be. Some of what Ashley describes could be outcomes if full human rights were realized for everyone but are not technically part of human rights ("harmony"). Yet, the important thing is that all these aspects were, in her mind, "basic." Through her listing of these aspects, she constructed an idealized image of human rights.

Serena, a SisterSong staff member, likened the human rights concept to the "backbone" of the reproductive justice movement. She explained,

The human rights framework, yeah, yeah, I mean you obviously know, but the human rights framework is the core. These are essential not only to American values, certainly, but to universal human values. These are core. Just the right to, the choice to. And then you fill in the blank, fill in the blank, fill in the blank, you know, fill in the blank. Whether it be economically, whether it be reproductively, whether it be environmentally, fill in the blank. But certainly I believe that it all is, it's all-encompassing. Human rights is all-encompassing. Reproductive justice is just a process that comes out of that framework. It's a part of. It's not a stand-alone issue, it's not stand-alone.[17]

Through her use of the "backbone" analogy, Serena demonstrates how the human rights framework holds together the reproductive justice movement. Further, she saw RJ as a "process"—not just a set of ideas that came from that framework. Thus, to separate the two was to, in her mind, incorrectly suggest that RJ was "stand-alone." These types of responses, along with others like Tonya's about grounding, provide examples of how interviewees conceptualize human rights as the "ground" or the base from which people can build a movement.

An Overarching Umbrella (Over)

Some interviewees conceptualized "human rights" as an overarching concept or set of rights that provided a source of protection. In this metaphor, human rights serve as an umbrella over a person.

This idea of an umbrella was supported by the reflections of interviewees such as Janel, an African American who worked for a national women's organization. She explained, "I just always, in my mind, figured that issues surrounding reproduction and reproductive freedom [were] definitely dictated on like rights that like every woman, essentially every person, is entitled to. So I guess in retrospect I was framing it under a human rights umbrella, but not knowingly."[18] This remark suggests that she is attempting to understand her own understanding. Without recalling key details, she had a vague sense of the existence of human rights.

Dera, a Black doula, answered my question about the definition of human rights in this way: "I think that somehow they're all intertwined, and I feel like human rights would be the umbrella, or I don't know, or human rights and like social justice would be the umbrella, possibly. But, I mean, at the same time I almost kinda feel like they're all on the same kinda plane, you know, 'cause it all deals with human beings and our rights and abilities to exercise and live and be free as human beings, you know, without somebody kinda impinging on that."[19] Dera's initial reference to a human rights "umbrella" suggests that human rights is a general concept that connotes overall protection that serves as a barrier against an external force. She elaborated to include social justice in this definition. She reconsiders this inclusion, unsure of its appropriateness, as indicated by "almost kinda feel." Yet, she is clear that these ideas are larger in scope.

A Thread Holding the Movement Together (Through)

A third common way that interviewees conceptualized human rights was as a connection, which I liken to a thread that joins pieces of fabric. Micaela, a Chicana based in Texas, noted early in our interview that she didn't hear people talking about "human rights." I inquired further. Then she noted the assumptions she makes when she does hear the phrase:

"What I see as human rights when I hear them like connecting all the rights together and stating it that they need to be connected together."[20]

"Wendy," a Black woman from Washington, DC, focused on the relationship between rights and autonomy: "I think *they're all intertwined.* I don't think that you can have human rights when you have women who are not in control of their own selves. You know, how can you have human rights when you have, you know, half your population being told what they can and cannot do?"[21] While she began by discussing the linkage between rights, she also included what she saw as a requirement for this interconnection to be real: control over one's self and one's decisions. This could raise doubt about the actual practice of human rights since in her answer she was reflecting on women's lack of control over their bodies. Yet, theoretically, she did see rights as connecting to each other.

Katherine, a reproductive rights lawyer, offered this reflection on the role of law in reproductive justice:

> And so I think what the reproductive justice movement [has done] . . . is broaden the discussions well beyond constitutional protections and *Roe,* and really focuses on human rights and the protections that are afforded through human rights, one of which being lack of discrimination . . . based on race and gender, so *incorporating* the two, . . . going back to intersectionalities, don't exist in the protection from the US court systems. And so I think that, you know, reproductive justice hasn't yet been a strong legal . . . thing because human rights really aren't recognized in this country.[22]

Katherine's point was that reproductive justice required connections between ideas and identities in ways that a narrow reproductive rights approach did not.

In this vein, a number of interviewees suggested that the most appealing part of a human rights framework was its ability to explain how individual concerns were embedded in broader structural relationships. Kierra Johnson, an African American woman who had begun her position as the executive director of a youth organization the week of our interview, explained, "The conversation around human rights allows us to, to go broader. . . . Um, it allows us to be specific about humanity and not make it about somebody's womb [laughter], you know what I mean? . . . I think it allows for us to, to really bring the whole person into the conversation."[23] Kierra's reflection may appear contradictory, but it points to the dynamic nature of human rights: broadening and specifying experiences. This dynamic is particularly important as various interviewees articulated feeling that their personal experiences were not easily categorized when analyzed through the singular lenses of race, gender, class, or sexuality. Instead, they advocated for the use of an intersectional framework when organizing their social movements, arguing that people's experiences meant that social movements needed to address the multiple origins of problems to solve those problems, thereby connecting different issues.

Human Rights as Similar yet Different from Social Justice

In an earlier chapter, I demonstrated how interviewees' linkage of "human rights" to "social justice" could be understood as a part of SisterSong's strategy of revolutionary domestication. However, at the time of their interviews, this linkage remained fluid for some interviewees. For example, Mehra reflected on her advocacy organization's transition: "I think that as an organization we believe that that shift is a conscious one and that we're obviously operating as an organization and in part of our mission we operate from part of this social justice/human rights angle."[24] Here was an explicit placing of the two as the same. Yet this interviewee also went on to differentiate her understandings of the concepts: "Ok, so 'human rights,' I think I always saw as 'international' and 'social justice' I think I saw as like *tangible ways that people are making a difference about human rights*."[25] She distinguished between the levels at which these ideas were operating. Social justice was "tangible," which implies that in contrast, "human rights" was not tangible. Therefore, since "human rights" as a concept felt abstract at times, "social justice" was necessary to bring in to localize this abstract concept.

Tonya, a Black woman who worked for a southern reproductive justice organization, recalled her exposure to various concepts: "I first really became interested and motivated by reproductive justice work by listening. I just happened to be in a space where social justice activists from the Gulf Coast had been working in the region. As far as the social justice, human rights activists, post-Katrina, which was the event which really galvanized or mobilized me into doing social justice work. I had been doing social justice–oriented work in academia as a part of a collective of Afro-descended scholars studying race and democracy in the Americas."[26] As she discussed the origins of her own advocacy, she slipped between the two ideas.

Taja, quoted earlier, seemed cautious about claiming knowledge about human rights:

> But I feel like RJ is kind of at the intersection. You know, we talk [about] an umbrella that's able to capture all these things. And if we were to draw a diagram, maybe it would be this complex web of intersections, and you find RJ in these particular places. Where it relates to the human rights framework, though, is where I'm not really able to really say much on because from a human rights perspective, I know very little about that. *I know more about social justice. Human rights has a more international implication. Social justice is a very US-used, you know, terminology and vocabulary. So I can speak from a social justice perspective.*[27]

She begins her definition of human rights using the "umbrella" framework. However, she later provides the caveat that she cannot speak to a relationship between concepts—then actually proceeds to do so. Responses like these offered an insight into people's fear of taking on the role of expert around issues about which they did not feel thoroughly familiar. Although their hesitance is understandable, I wondered whether it impeded their ability to take on the role that some SisterSong leaders wanted for them, namely, as human rights advocates.

Maame-Mensima, quoted earlier, described her work in the following way: "We do a lot of bringing people together, and we do a lot of training. So, helping people understand how the reproductive justice framework can be used in the work that they do and *human rights and social justice work*, which is important because . . . me being where I am in my life, I realized how much my reproduction is impacted by so much around me."[28] Maame-Mensima's statement served as further indication of how important it was to have continual exposure to concepts such as human rights in order to reinforce them. As noted earlier, Maame-

Mensima's upbringing meant that she had exposure to a range of issues in the global sphere and already had exposure to ideas of human rights. Yet her understanding was enhanced through her continued interaction with other people as she helped them understand this idea. Further, her comment exposed the way discussing the intricacies of how human rights affected an arena salient to her current concerns—reproduction— reinforced her understanding of the importance of human rights in other arenas.

Kendra, who worked in the Midwest on issues of sexual violence, learned about SisterSong when we participated in the United Nations Commission on the Status of Women, and I told the group about my research. At the time, she had looked at the SisterSong website and been interested. A year later, one of the organizations with which Kendra was affiliated brought in Ross as a keynote speaker. At Ross's request, her visit included a meeting that Kendra described as a "Reproductive Justice 101 seminar for women of color." Kendra reflected on the meeting and Ross's public talk:

> There needs to be a refocus on how those things interact, and I think that Loretta's on the right track when she talks about human rights, right, that the human rights–based approach, I think, will be useful in reframing these things, right, or looking at ways to increase the power of this movement. So I think that my number one kind of thing is that a movement needs to emerge that talks about the lack of cultural awareness and validation of social justice work. I think it's the first point that needs to be talked about. So like kids like in elementary school and stuff need to be taught about social justice and about their responsibility as a citizen to, you know, like know what's going on in their communities and to know, you know, that if something's not right, that it's not only their choice but their responsibility to kinda make it right.[29]

This response held several complex ideas. Kendra clearly knew there was something different about the two concepts. In her mind, there was the clear association between "human rights" and SisterSong's coordinator. This interviewee identified Ross most closely with promoting human rights and moving down a "track" with it, so to speak.

On the other hand, she quickly moved between discussion of human rights and discussion of social justice. She then noted the importance of teaching children collective obligation. This latter discussion gets at the role of cultural change being critical. Kendra attended SisterSong's Let's Talk About Sex! conference in Miami the next year.

A number of interviewees articulated the potential for social justice to feel more concrete. Ashley, a White college student in the Midwest, reflected, "I think of reproductive justice more so in the way that I think of social justice, which is the active fight toward ensuring that human rights are, that human rights are being protected, and that making, you know, making sure that individuals and corporations and governing bodies respect those human rights of people. And, you know, doing it inside and outside of like the governmental systems. So not just lobbying, but also doing grassroots work within communities, like setting up healthcare units or, you know, educating young people about their rights."[30] Ashley differentiated levels at which to engage in social change: there was work "inside" institutions, like lobbying, and work "outside" institutions, like "grassroots work within communities," which involved creating community services and educating people. Her emphasis on social justice requiring "active" efforts suggests that, in her mind, human rights existed but required effort to achieve.

Dessa, a White, Michigan-based organizer, considered the different ways she used terms:

> I think about "social justice" more than I do about "human rights." I mean I think about human rights, but I use the term "social justice" a lot more often. So I mean I can hear myself saying like "abortion as an option is a human right" because it's your body, and what is more fundamental of a thing to your right over than your own body? And since I believe healthcare is a human right, that falls into there, too. I use "social justice" a lot because I don't, I mean I personally don't just care about reproductive justice. I care about environmental justice and civil rights and other stuff, LGBT rights, immigration rights, all those things that really have a lot to do with reproduction in so many ways.[31]

When I asked her to expand on her answer, she offered an answer like Ashley's:

I guess like reproductive rights would be based more on laws, and when I think of human rights, I think of these basic things that are kind of inalienable, water, food, shelter, education, healthcare, democracy. I think of it more in like a legal framework, and maybe what governments should be doing for their people. And then I guess when I think of the justice, I think about how it all intertwines and how it works as a community, and how things affect each other beyond what just a government can provide or just what law is there to protect those things.

Thus, while "human rights" and "social justice" were related in Dessa's mind, the former emphasized a relationship between a government and its people while the latter went farther to also include relationships *between* people.

Integrating Human Rights

While there were varying frameworks for conceptualizing human rights, I want to highlight one set of interviewees, the integrators, a small but meaningful number of interviewees. On the opposite end of the spectrum from skeptics were integrators who, contrary to others' perception of human rights as abstract, thought that a human rights framework was crucial motivation because it provided a concrete way to interpret domestic social problems. Integrators differed from learners due to their discussion of incorporating human rights into their lives and using the concept as an everyday framework. They understood human rights as highly relevant to their daily lives, and used them as guidelines for how to proceed in the world. For them, human rights provide both a goal to work toward and the motivation needed to perform often emotionally draining work.

Serena, a SisterSong staffer, explained her approach to teaching a college communications class: "Now that it's come full circle, now I'm teaching college students, there's no way in hell I could do anything I do in class—in regards of teaching public speaking—and them not understand human rights, them not understanding oppressions because I tell them the first day of class, you will not, I will not tolerate, I won't tolerate, you will not be permitted to oppress anybody in my class in your speeches. . . . So we talk about intersectionality and we talk about human rights and we talk about social justice issues."[32] Here she clearly identified individuals as able to violate human rights.

Like Serena, Tonya also wanted to teach human rights within a classroom setting. Unfortunately, she found it difficult to acquire texts that discussed human rights in a US context: "I'm teaching the first class on human rights theory and practice at the university . . . which is a challenge because it's difficult to even find a text which centers US experience within that." Tonya had knowledge, which as noted earlier had initially come from international advocacy work, but when trying to apply it to the United States in a formal way, she had trouble doing so. This is not too surprising, though, since, again, restrictive domestication by the US government results in few public models for human rights education.

La' Tasha, the aforementioned executive director of a Pittsburgh-based reproductive justice organization, explained part of her progression in thinking about human rights and her relationship to SisterSong, in which she was increasingly active. She elucidated,

> Human rights, I think, has been kind of framed as out . . . not in here, in this country, not here in the United States. And you know, I can honestly say before a year ago that . . . that I probably thought that too, but there are human rights and justices right here in my neighborhood, you know what I mean? And . . . and like for instance, women in Philadelphia and Pittsburgh organizing to make sure that pregnant women . . . incarcerated women who are pregnant don't have to give birth shackled. That's a human rights injustice. So yes, my own personal framework has definitely changed.[33]

La' Tasha identified how, prior to her involvement with SisterSong, she had understood human rights in the common way restrictive domestication produces: "not here in the United States." But now she could see that human rights problems indeed existed "in my neighborhood." Her statement indicates how the distance between human rights and herself shifted. The shift was not only seeing human rights violation as happening here, in a broad sense in the United States. Rather, they were very close to her as she went about her daily life.

The importance of distance came up in the interview of another integrator, "Inez," a Latina/Native American doula in the Midwest. She volunteered with an organization that was transitioning to a reproductive justice approach. The RJ 101 workshop she attended influenced her view of human rights: "I think that . . . probably the most concrete information that I gleaned from the Reproductive Justice 101 training was the way that Loretta [Ross] talked about the human rights framework and broke down kind of oppression and human rights and very specific human rights issues."[34] She explained how human rights provided her family guidance through ritual:

And recently my wife and I bought a poster . . . with the International Declaration of Human Rights [on it]. . . . We have an eight-year-old, and that's what we read before we eat dinner now [laughs]. . . . I'll be at a birth that's really traumatic and where a woman is not treated well, or I feel like it's a lot of trauma from it myself, and I need to know that there's some kinda concrete something that, at the end of the day, defines where my values are and what I'm trying to achieve. 'Cause sometimes it seems so impossible. It seems so stretched out and all over the place. That's like our blessing for dinner, that this is what we're going for in the household and beyond.[35]

Rather than viewing human rights in an abstract manner, Inez articulated feeling that the importance of human rights was reinforced for her every day. First, she discussed interpreting an experience she witnessed as a human rights violation. Then, she used a human rights lens to transform the experience into a source of inspiration to remind her why human rights *are* needed. Finally, Inez discussed how she and her family "consume" human rights by putting a human rights poster in a location they see regularly and integrating it into their dinner routine.[36] The poster provided them a consistent reminder of the range of human rights and what a world with human rights would look like. Inez literally brought human rights home into *her* domestic sphere, where she taught a future generation how to give human rights the respect she felt they deserved.

Human rights learners, described earlier in the chapter, may integrate socially progressive practices into their lives, but unlike the handful of integrators, they do not consciously identify human rights as the motivation of their participation in these practices. Many interviewees' involvement in activities to improve their local and/or national community would be evidence of exemplary socially just activities, but integrators' identification of the origin or continued participation in those activities as related to human rights differentiates them from most interviewees.

A common assumption among people who call for change in the United States is that activists from various progressive movements will play a central role in creating this new culture. Accordingly, "The idea is that once well-entrenched in local culture, human rights will be part of the ethical lens through which the problems in society are refracted. . . . To put it plainly, the general public must 'buy into' the values promoted by human rights and agree to support the mechanisms designed to advance those values."[37] Yet, because human rights are "alternatively approached as a philosophical idea, a legal concept, or a political project,"[38] they can be understood in many ways even among the people who are assumed to support them wholeheartedly (i.e., progressive activists).

This chapter provides us a lens into a liminal category of rights consciousness because human rights consciousness in the United States is an example of an otherwise legal consciousness that must develop without institutional support (e.g., courts). In many cases outside of social movement rallies (and even in them), it is still not the norm to claim injustice in terms of a human rights violation because the history of the United States differs from that of other Western powers that have recognized a spectrum of human rights. To speak generally about rights consciousness would be incorrect in the case of all types of rights. While some of the themes from my data are like others found in prior research, other themes offer new ways to consider the role of human rights in movement participants' lives.

Theorists suggest that legal consciousness can be produced in everyday relationships to the law because law "operates through social life as persons and groups deliberately interpret and invoke law's language, authority, and procedures to organize their lives and manage their relationships."[39] However, if, as Ewick and Silbey proposed decades ago, legal consciousness emerges from an iterative process, this process would seem largely absent in the case of human rights in the United States because human rights are not part of most US residents' initial sense of law. On the commonness of law, Ewick and Silbey presume that people maintain a level of familiarity with law—not a mastery, per se, but some level of familiarity. In their daily lives, people continually engage with the law whether through formal legal procedures, mass media, or even conversations. Thus, "In short, the commonplace operation of law in daily life makes us all legal agents insofar as we actively make law, even when no formal legal agent is involved."[40] Their conceptualization of legality assumes intentionality ("deliberately") and agency ("actively") even in the absence of formal law.

Again, there is limited evidence—or engagement on this level—with human rights. They conceptualize two key features of law: its being remote, which is true of human rights, as I show above, and its being a game.[41] The latter, the "game" feature, does not apply in the case of human right because many people don't even know there is a "game," let alone how to find the directions, how to read the directions, and therefore how to play. For SMOs trying to engage human rights, this all points to a dim picture of limited possibilities for leveraging human rights discourse. Many interviewees' reflections offer a "common sense" understanding of human rights versus formal learning that can occur in law school. As studies show, many people are *not* aware of such a thing as human rights although they are aware of the US legal system, with which they have many interactions (through personal experience, popular media, etc.).

Interviewees like Lucie who had learned about human rights early are a different model for integration since she learned early to assume she had a right to human rights. This could therefore provide a basis of a worldview or understanding of herself as valuable and human. She differed from other integrator interviewees who eventually learned about human rights as something that they had a right to demand. Yet, the possibility lies in the insight that comes from looking at later integrators: *feeling* human rights experientially allowed them to connect the dots. This shows the potential of experiential learning in creating a successful human rights–based reproductive justice movement.

8

"Puppies and Rainbows" or Pragmatic Politics?

Organizations Engaging with Human Rights

Between the two periods in which I conducted interviews, Senator Barack Obama became the United States' first African American president with continued appeals to "change" and "hope." A range of groups, both in support of and in opposition to Obama's election in 2008, were confident that his election would produce a drastic change in the United States' approach to foreign and domestic policy. However, while a new president shifts the political landscape and Obama's election signaled change in some ways, the US government's activity around human rights remained "ambivalent," to use a generous phrase offered by one scholar to describe the US government's earlier approach to human rights.[1]

For progressive activists, there were signs that he would engage with the United Nations in earnest. For example, in 2009, for the first time in years, the United States sent a delegation to the United Nations 53rd Commission on the Status of Women (CSW), a two-week meeting in New York attended by government delegations and thousands of nongovernmental organizations (NGOs, generally SMOs). I participated in the CSW as a member of the Practicum in Advocacy at the United Nations, sponsored jointly by the Women's International League for Peace and Freedom, the National Women's Studies Association, and Suffolk University. While I do not have access to any instructions US delegates received regarding their participation, they did not appear to be at the CSW simply for "show" or to disrupt the process, which contrasts with the way more conservative administrations previously participated in the UN meetings.[2] An example of constructive engagement with the UN was that for the first time ever, the US government's delegation held multiple informal briefings for US NGOs. At these sessions, the US delegates discussed their commitment to women's rights, fielded questions about the Obama administration's stance on issues such as ratification of the Convention on the Elimination of Discrimination Against Women (CEDAW), and attempted to reassure the audience that the Obama administration would take human rights seriously. While attending one of these informal NGO briefings, we invited one of the US delegates to speak to our group. She agreed and the next morning over breakfast fielded questions from our group on concerns such as rape as a weapon of war and inconsistencies between US global and domestic reproductive health policy.

As another example of constructive engagement with the UN, the Obama administration government submitted to its first Universal Periodic Review (UPR) starting in 2010. The United Nations designed the UPR in 2006. The months-long process involves a nation reporting on its human rights records and consulting with NGOs, representatives from three randomly selected countries reviewing the record, a public defense of the record, receipt of recommendations, and a formal written response to the recommendations. These actions, among others, seemed to signify that the US government was moving towards supporting a range of human rights. This would theoretically, in turn, help foster a supportive human rights culture in which people understood human rights and the Universal Declaration of Human Rights as the standard they expect the US government to uphold.

While the Obama administration engaged in the UPR process, the administration's formal response disappointed many activists. In the initial report, the government began by explaining its goals for the report: "We present our first Universal Periodic Review (UPR) report in the context of our commitment to help to build a world in which universal rights give strength and direction to the nations, partnerships, and institutions that can usher us toward a more perfect world, a world characterized by, as President Obama has said, 'a just peace based on the inherent rights and dignity of every individual.'"[3] Noticeably, the administration's "commitment" was to building a world with "universal rights," not "universal human rights." This is a small difference in wording, but since this report specifically focused on the US government's human rights record, it is a noticeable omission. Thus, by not being consistently specific, the US government was leaving rights open to interpretation. Perhaps the administration was tempering an embrace of human rights?

This could be the case, but the government's later documents make clear that the Obama administration would only move so far on human rights as understood globally.

As with some other United Nations processes, NGOs submitted unofficial "shadow" reports about the status of human rights issues. Over twenty reports were submitted on topics ranging from corporate accountability to migrant labor. A number of reports discussed health, including one colloquially referred to as the "reproductive rights" report. SisterSong and six other organizations submitted this report, formally titled the "Report on the United States' Compliance with Its Human Rights Obligations in the Area of Women's Reproductive and Sexual Health." As with most organizations, all of the members of each organization did not vote on the report language. Rather, key leaders engaged in the drafting. The report summarized "three areas of reproductive rights that treaty monitoring bodies have identified as issues of human rights concern: (1) pervasive racial disparities in reproductive and sexual health; (2) obstacles to women's access to safe, legal abortion; and (3) the practice of shackling incarcerated pregnant women."[4] The report outlined various health disparities and made the case that the US government needed to protect abortion providers as "human rights defenders." Referring to abortion as a human right was not new, but casting abortion providers as human rights defenders was a reframing. Further, the linking of abortion access and incarcerated women's pregnancy would not seem an obvious choice to people focusing on traditional reproductive rights issues. Thus, the influence of reproductive justice advocates is clear with this inclusion.

A 2010 *Wall Street Journal* editorial about the UPR argued that the "cause of human rights has been systematically corrupted."[5] The argument was based on the idea that the US government participating in the UPR and lauding itself for its support of human rights domestically tacitly supported corruption since nations that regularly violate human rights could still participate in the UPR. This editorial in a highly visible media forum meant that the public's exposure to human rights was in a negative representation. Public denunciations such as these add a challenge for movements trying to promote human rights since they must first overcome the negativity bias. But the *WSJ* need not have worried about the Obama administration legitimating human rights. The

US government responded to the recommendations, then offered a second qualified response to clarify its prior language:

> What it means for a recommendation to "enjoy our support" needs explanation. Some recommendations ask us to achieve an ideal, e.g., end discrimination or police brutality, and others request action not entirely under the control of our Federal Executive Branch, e.g., adopt legislation, ratify particular treaties, or take action at the state level. Such recommendations enjoy our support, or enjoy our support in part, when we share the ideal that the recommendations express, are making serious efforts toward achieving their goals, and intend to continue to do so. *Nonetheless, we recognize, realistically, that the United States may never completely accomplish what is described in the literal terms of the recommendation.* We are also comfortable supporting a recommendation to do something that we already do, and intend to continue doing, without in any way implying that we agree with a recommendation that understates the success of our ongoing efforts.[6]

In a simultaneously simple and convoluted clarification, the Obama administration essentially acknowledged the recommendations and offered abstract support for many of them. At the same time, the Obama administration clarified that (1) various UPR recommendations were unrealistic considering the United States' multilayered government and (2) the government would proceed with its current course of action. In sum, the status quo would remain.

The United States' official dual response of support and dismissiveness disappointed advocates. One *Huffington Post* columnist commented, "This acceptance was primarily rhetorical, pointing to *existing laws and commitments. The government missed the opportunity to legitimize its vague promises with concrete policy commitments and actions.* While rhetorical support for human rights has its role, it is imperative that every government ensures that people can enjoy these rights in their day-to-day lives. Yet the U.S. government has actively undermined—even in its actions over recent weeks and months—the very recommendations on economic and social rights it purports to support."[7] The columnist provided a cogent analysis but failed in one major respect: claiming that the US government had "missed the opportunity," which suggests an unintentional or unforeseeable consequence of its actions. Rather, as I have argued, the US government has consistently engaged in restrictive domestication: a concerted effort over decades to limit the meaning of human rights and interpret them to fit its own priorities. As noted by the columnist, the government's priorities are visible in existing practices. Thus, the Obama administration's response was characteristic.

The editorial fits into a tradition human rights practitioners have engaged for decades: "The most well-known tactic of human rights civil society has been that of 'naming, blaming and shaming,' that is naming human rights violations, publicly identifying the violator (tradition-ally a state but increasingly a corporation or other actor), and shaming them into compliance by employing a public campaign (involving letter writing and other public acts of condemnation)."[8] Another way to put this would be to say that human rights advocates "call out" a govern-ment for how the government fails to live up to human rights stan-dards. As simple as this tactic seems, it is limited by how amenable an administration is to those claims. Advocates use this tactic in a range of nations, but it is more difficult to deploy in the United States due to the government's self-professed and documented exceptionalism. When it comes to the US government, there is no broad "shame" to induce—US exceptionalism creates a narrative of superiority and righteousness of action.

For example, Senator John Kerry, in his role on the Senate Foreign Relations Committee, discussed supporting a UN disability treaty. He invoked the idea of the United States as a global leader. Kerry, accord-ing to an article by Jim Abrams, "'said the impact of the treaty will echo around the world,'" further noting that "he [Kerry] said the Americans with Disabilities Act [ADA] is the gold standard for protecting the rights of the disabled and the treaty would 'take that gold standard and ex-tend it to countries that have never heard of disability rights.' He said that it would benefit disabled American veterans who want to travel or work abroad."[9] This article offers a good description of US exceptional-ism. Various US civil rights advocates would note that the ADA may be a "gold standard," but there is still extensive struggle to ensure basic compliance. The example offered of a person who could be affected by disability was a veteran, like Kerry, a "deserving" citizen with whom leg-islators would be likely to sympathize. This is an example of how the US government focuses on expanding its model to others, whether or not its view of a social issue and approach (e.g., civil rights protection) is the way other countries operate.

During Obama's presidency there was also the contradictory reality that publicly he appeared more willing than many other presidents to talk about social issues (e.g., race relations, as demonstrated by his 2008 campaign speech "A More Perfect Union") and attempt to make changes that would benefit a wide range of people (e.g., the Affordable Care Act that ushered in healthcare reform). Still, these changes all occurred within a capitalist, neoliberal economic model and admonishments of "personal responsibility" that characterized previous administrations.[10] Thus, Obama's actions loosened the tightness of restrictive domestication in one arena, but the possibility of expanding US citizens' rights to a range of economic and social rights was not a foregone conclusion. He still championed a specific economic model.

Unsurprisingly, then, few US organizations engage with human rights discourse in the domestic arena, even if they have "human rights" in their title. One example is Human Rights Campaign (HRC). In her research, Fetner describes HRC as a "multi-issue group primarily concerned with anti-discrimination legislation for lesbians and gay men, reform of sodomy laws, increased funding for women's health concerns and AIDS research and treatment."[11] More recently, HRC described itself as "an organization that dedicates itself to equality for gay, lesbian, bisexual, and transgender people."[12] HRC's website makes no mention of the origin of the phrase "human rights," provides no explanation of the Universal Declaration of Human Rights, and offers no discussion of human rights organizing around LGBT rights in international politics. Further, the logo is the mathematical "equal" sign, which hints at civil rights—equality under the law. While equality is important, it is partial. That concept fails to recognize that different groups can live in equally dismal conditions but still not have their human rights— thereby experiencing equality under the law, but not experiencing flourishing. Thus, while Human Rights Campaign and similar organizations invoking the notion of human rights engage in activities that help create a more just society, these organizations do not link their work to a history of human rights activism, and most have only recently begun to discuss working in the global arena.

Due to "discomfort" with seeming unreasonable, "even staunch supporters of civil and political rights may regard economic and social rights as better suited to a letter to Santa Claus," leading them to pursue restrictive approaches.[13] Thus, it is interesting, and rare, when a social movement organization discusses human rights with attention to international and domestic relevance and the range of human rights.

Moving from Abstract Values to Concrete Connections

There were a variety of ways interviewees discussed the practicality of "human rights," which hinged on organizations' leaders' understanding of how their multiple audiences—their own members, the public, legislators—understood the concept. Kierra, the executive director of Choice USA (now URGE), a national pro-choice youth organization that was a SisterSong affiliate, noted the difficulty in translating "human rights":

> I mean it's, it's us really trying to, to move from the concept to the practical application. And so for us, it's trying to figure out how do we practically relate people back to that [human rights] in a way that doesn't just fit . . . in kind of cyberspace . . . on our website. . . . [W]e had our strategic planning, like a couple years ago, and we're constantly in this process of changing our language to reflect, you know, what our values are, and being that human rights is one of those, it's us trying to figure out, again, like how to make sure all of our materials and organizing and our workshops reflect that.[14]

Kierra's reflection demonstrates how even in an organizational setting where staff abstractly support human rights, translating support into concrete organizational practices requires effort. Essentially, social movement organizations must make a conscious effort to link their publicly stated values to programs and practices. To go beyond language in "cyberspace" (where organizations post mission statements) requires consistently evaluating how to enact human rights. Otherwise, "human rights" evokes little meaning to the people for whom organizations advocate.

Aimee Thorne-Thomsen, the Latina executive director of the Pro-Choice Public Education Project (PEP), a SisterSong affiliate organization, explained the considerations around using human rights:

> Well, you know, it's kind of funny in that the word "rights," just from our work, is problematic. And not necessarily expressing human rights, but we've seen that people, again, from our research and our work, people take rights for granted. You know, like one of the reasons "reproductive rights" as a term doesn't resonate with a lot of people is 'cause people assume they have rights. So like, there's nothing to really fight for or get all, you know, worked up about because, you know, this is a right, it's a done deal. Never mind that, you know, civil rights and abortion rights and all that stuff aren't quite settled. But there's this sense that rights are settled, you don't have to keep fighting for them, they're there when I want them. And that's part of our history coming from a sort of traditional pro-choice movement.

Aimee identified a general problem with the idea of "rights"—a sense of their being settled—which then affected possibilities for a discussion of rights, human or otherwise. Beyond being an issue of language, the perception of rights as settled affected possibilities for mobilization. If rights were settled, then people had no reason to be concerned about protecting them. As she points out, this is not the reality of rights, but can be people's *perception* of rights.

On human rights specifically, her answer hinted at the consequences of the government's restrictive domestication:

> Our awareness of human rights was really late and slow. And thinking about sort of how to translate that to the U.S., which is so self-centered and doesn't believe it has, like, anything in common with anyone else has been challenging. . . . I think that what we've taken from the human rights framework is really this sense that as human beings, we have—and this is the way we use "the rights"—if you will, is we have the right to live healthy lives within our families, within our communities, you know, within ourselves. And so we've sort of tried to demystify it and use really plain language to kind of talk about some of the issues we face, and to talk about the interconnectedness of them.[15]

Aimee speaks to "translating" specific human rights ideas into "plain language." Plain language is used to illuminate both oppression ("issues") and an ultimate vision ("healthy lives"). Of course, audiences vary on what they want in order to achieve that vision, but her point was that when considering human rights, her organization needed to consider the US government's history, the assumptions audiences bring when engaging with the organization (e.g., rights as settled), and how to help bridge the gap between those understandings and a vision of the future the organization needed people to be excited enough about to take action to bring it to fruition.

Some interviewees also noted how the more they learned about reproductive justice, the more attention they paid to human rights and its implications for organizational practice. Zarah, with a Chicago-based youth organization, reflected on these shifts:

> And when I was at SisterSong [conference] in, not, last year, listening to Loretta Ross talk about it being a human right, it being reproductive justice framework, being based off of the human rights framework. Shifted us once again, right. 'Cause that's not knowledge that we were initially privy to when we first started talking about being a reproductive justice organization. I mean, being an extension of is, I think there's new, and I don't know the right language, but there's new committees talking about sexuality as a human right. . . . And so in our society, reproductive justice and rights often being deemed as "oh, a woman's issue." When you present it as a human rights issue people can't deny certain things. It makes it an easier conversation to have on the whole. Young women have a right to live in a community free of toxins that won't determine, won't be the dictator of whether they can physically bear children or not.

She was not seeing human rights as a moral issue. Rather, human rights was just what is. In our society, they come under a banner of morality, which makes it difficult to make progress on them. She saw embracing human rights as eventually solving opposition to specific "women's issues" by moving the issues to the purview of unmarked "humans."

Another way interviewees considered human rights positively was in the discourse's ability to facilitate organizations connecting with each other. Charlene, a Chicana cofounder of a Latina reproductive health organization, reflected on her decades in the field. She noted, "So I actually think that that's one way that we can connect the dots when we talk about human rights versus reproductive health rights, you know, reproductive health and reproductive rights, because I think that if we just talk about fundamental human rights then folks who are working in environmental justice, we can connect there, because it is a basic human right to have these kinds of things no matter where you live on this universe, you know. And so when we talk about it there, that's how we can then partner with different folks."[16] Her discussion of human rights focused on how the idea serves as a connector. Beyond connecting people, it expanded relationships between organizations, creating possibilities for coalition. Charlene's seemingly hyperbolic reference to "this universe" shows an expansive vision of human rights.

The Ambiguous Relationship between Human Rights and Social Justice

As discussed in a prior chapter, at various points in data collection, I came across many examples of the slippage between "human rights" and "social justice." Yet, some interviewees explicated the conscious choice to move *between* those ideas and the logics for doing so. One interviewee, a White woman named Moira, coordinated some programming for Asian Communities for Reproductive Justice (ACRJ):

> I mean ACRJ has always been firmly placed, has always placed itself within the social justice movement. So especially at the local and statewide level, we are in close relationship to a broad range of social justice groups, from racial justice groups to immigrant rights groups to workers' rights groups to youth justice groups to education justice groups. Like that's where we see reproductive justice fit: is in the social justice movement. We're also very well aware . . . of the linkages and the interplay between reproductive justice in the United States and the human rights framework more globally. And we find that it's especially useful in terms of talking about the affirmative role of government in ensuring reproductive justice for community. . . . [W]e most often use the language of 'social justice' rather than 'human rights' in terms of when we're, you know, in our organizing program and in our collective projects. But more and

more, especially as we talk about sort of Strong Families and sort of the policy needs that are necessary to support strong families and reproductive justice, that the framework of human rights is critical in providing groundwork for that.[17]

Here, Moira used "social justice" more and discussed the range of social justice movements in which she saw ACRJ and the reproductive justice movement embedded. Yet, she also cited recognition of a *global* human rights movement, although that is not where she specifically places the RJ movement, since it has "linkages" to (rather than being embedded in) a global movement. In explaining the utility of "human rights" in a specific campaign (Strong Families), Moira showed how organizations could shift. As in a prior chapter, we also see human rights conceptualized as providing a ground or foundation for specific action ("groundwork").

Challenges to Using Human Rights

In this section I discuss a few challenges that interviewees discussed regarding trying to engage with the concept of human rights. These challenges came down to two main areas: elite power brokers' hostility and audiences' misunderstanding of human rights.

One interviewee reflected on her organization's reticence to explicitly use a human rights frame as being connected to concerns about legal regimes:

> We definitely adopt like reproductive health and rights as like, you know, human rights. But we definitely don't use, we don't use that term. I mean, I think it's more so because like, the organization fears that like, reproductive justice would kinda like, it kind of reeks of like, the judicial system. *And the organization fears that like the general public would kinda like misconstrue the concept of making that leap of reproductive justice and human rights, and confound it with like, the Supreme Court, you know.* I think that's pretty much the only reason why we don't use the term. But we definitely are on that bandwagon ideologically.[18]

Gina's remark offers an interesting example of how different concepts overlap in ways that can limit how organizations choose to frame their work. She suggests that there is a possibility of audiences connecting reproductive justice and human rights to the US legal system. She goes so far as to say "reeks," which is a negative term that evokes disgust. A perceived connection to a legal system could taint human rights. Gina articulated concerns about audiences connecting human rights to the Supreme Court. While human rights are not specifically protected by the Supreme Court, this was her guess as to potential audiences' approach.

Later in the interview she gave examples of how the organization did explicitly connect its advocacy efforts with human rights by having a program on International Human Rights Day (celebrated annually on December 10). However, in her view, despite the organization doing activities connected to formal human rights celebrations, they explicitly chose to not talk about "human rights" due to audiences potentially assuming a legal connection. Her answer highlights a few things: the lack of clarity around the legal status of human rights in the United States and the organization's need to balance its values with audience knowledge—or perceived knowledge—of an issue.

Some interviewees had different ways of articulating the challenge of doing more to bring human rights within their organizational spaces. Their perspective was based on their involvement with organizations that work around reproductive health and rights advocacy rather than reproductive justice, per se. As discussed earlier, these two approaches focus on access to and provision of reproductive health but not necessarily broad social transformation, which reproductive justice advocates generally see as their larger goal.

One interviewee spoke at length about the impracticality of human rights discourse when trying to sway specific audiences, namely, people with power. "Karin," an African American/Latina with a reproductive health organization, reflected on the role of human rights in national policy advocacy that occurred on "the Hill," as she termed it. Candidly, she said, "Right now we are in a pragmatist environment politically. So whatever works. And so it's kind of a 'know your audience.' And so if we're talking to a very liberal member who's super, super lefty and all of that, and you wanna talk puppies and rainbows and human rights and whatever. . . . [I]t's very sad that human rights is puppies and rainbows [laughs]. . . . [But] we're thinking, you know, in very much more practical terms."[19] Karin's initial reflection focused on pragmatics. When activists are trying to pass legislation, human rights–related arguments are likely to be seen as impractical and idealistic. Her laughter indicated an acknowledgment that this should not be the way human rights are viewed ("it's very sad"). However, this is the reality of a "pragmatic environment politically" that requires continual compromise. Alternative frames such as economic efficiency had greater power to persuade legislators—and voters—of all political parties. While Karin's logic makes sense from the perspective of passing policy, there is a drawback. Discussing human rights in a policy context is only useful with people who are already somewhat knowledgeable or at least supportive of human rights. Yet, this creates a tautological situation: if people who are already receptive to some version of human rights are the only ones with whom activists talk about human rights, these same people may remain the only ones supporting human rights.

Our interview occurred in Washington, DC, while legislators literally debated nuances of the Affordable Care Act, President Obama's proposal for a nationalized healthcare system. Karin continued discussing the balance of considerations for gaining political support and why "human rights" was not as useful in her work:

> So we don't have to figure out if we're gonna make it left or leftier, right. [laughing] That's not, that's not the debate is, "Are we gonna use RJ or human rights?" [laughing] Like that's not the question. The question is are we gonna talk, in terms of pragmatism, are we gonna use, you know, an economic argument. . . . And so in terms of *our* issues what is gonna appeal to, you know, middle or conservative . . . are you talking national security, are you talking economics, are you talking like, so like those kind of base issues like immigration. So what is the overlay of our issues with those issues? And so it's really scary because when you're talking about family planning as a cost-saver, you know.[20]

Based on her experience, Karin thought that focusing on familiar ideas of economic efficiency had greater power to persuade legislators of all political parties. An example of this type of argument includes pointing to studies that show that the government investing in contraceptive access now saves taxpayers money in the future.[21] The implication is that essentially, preventing low-income people's pregnancy now prevents having to pay for social services for their children in the future. However, reproductive justice activists find economic arguments abhorrent due to their proximity to eugenic thinking. Arguments about cost savings place value on certain communities *not* reproducing, such as teenagers or people using Medicaid insurance. The argument for access is not based on commitment to the human right to control family size or human health, but rather cost savings, which at best can be traced to frugality and at worst, eugenics. Further, economic arguments rarely address the fact that even people defined as middle-class increasingly struggle to care for their children due to the rising cost of housing and changing economic structures that have reduced the types of jobs that offer basic healthcare.

Karin offered a bleaker picture than she had painted initially when she pointed to the consequences she saw of restrictive domestication—the US government restricting the meaning of human rights to civil and political rights. With two courses of action being to talk about human rights and potentially alienate some tenuous allies or not to talk about human rights and reduce the risk of alienation, pragmatic politics can undermine broader approaches, irrespective of one's own personal interest in human rights promotion.

Her emphasis on pragmatism makes sense considering the US policymaking structure. One of the most-cited theories on policymaking emphasizes that issues have to first appear on an agenda before policymaking occurs.[22] Even after there is a sense that there is an "an idea whose time has come," policymaking involves three separate yet related streams: the political stream, the problem stream (agreement that the issue constitutes a problem worthy of solving), and the policy stream.[23] Policy change requires convergence of two streams, and for a policy window to open. Thus, many processes and actors must align. The US legislative process leaves little room for alternative frameworks and requires such a level of maneuvering and forecasting that taking risks appears illogical. Framing issues in terms of human rights remains one of those risks and, as interviewees such as Karin demonstrate, can appear a naïve proposition. But this was in tension with the way some SisterSong leaders wanted policy work to proceed. Reflecting on a common problem with policy advocacy, Ross noted, "I'm not gonna come home from Washington [DC] saying 'we got a bill [legislation] through but, I'm sorry, we had to sell you out to do it." I mean you don't build movement that way, in my mind, particularly if your movement is supposed to center the most vulnerable people in the center of the lens. They aren't the first people you lop off, you know, unless you're pimping them. But if you're really representing them, you have to do it differently." Ross highlighted the difference between policy advocacy that centered "vulnerable people" and policy advocacy that exploited them.[24]

Particularly illustrative of this tension were the lobbying efforts that occurred during SisterSong's November 2009 membership meeting titled "The Color of Power: Voices for Change." Policy was a focus of the meeting, as indicated by the description (SisterSong Fifth Annual National Membership Meeting & Advocacy Day), the location (Washington, DC), and the scheduling of the advocacy/lobbying day for the Monday after the conference. As it happened, legislators were debating the Affordable Care Act (i.e., healthcare reform) during the conference. As I discuss elsewhere, this shifted the tenor and plans for the conference.[25]

On the morning of a Saturday membership meeting in November 2009 in Washington, DC, the leadership announced that it had learned that the Stupak Amendment—which aimed to restrict abortion within the proposed Affordable Care Act—would probably be discussed on the floor that day.[26] At the mention of a possible march, most of the couple of hundred people in the room stood up, clapping in support. Later, leadership presented possible options that included proceeding with the conference as planned, holding a press conference, conducting lobby visits with individual legislators, waiting on a permit to march to the Capitol, and marching to the Capitol without a permit and risking arrest. The final option received wide applause. After some conference attendees began to move to a different room to make signs for the march, the presentation continued with an explanation of the risks of marching without a permit. While protesting without a permit risks arrest throughout the United States, the District of Columbia is under federal jurisdiction, with generally harsher consequences. Any undocumented women in attendance could try to participate and leave before reaching the main area patrolled by police, but they, like anyone else, could be arrested at any time. The difference, however, was that undocumented women could also face deportation.

Based on the exclamations of "Oh!" that arose in the room, many people had not considered the presence of or implications for undocumented women. While the gender and race of US women of color place them in subordinated categories, women of color with citizenship can take for granted certain privileges. While we know protest actions by people of color receive greater scrutiny,[27] people of color with US citizenship have little fear of permanent separation from their country of residence.

As this instance highlighted, the "sisterhood" of women of color can reach across borders, but only some women can be assured of their right to return across those borders. Despite the various efforts to emphasize only a collective identity as women of color with a shared fate, other intragroup differences are politically salient. As in the case of immigration status, to facilitate the participation of *all* women of color, the myriad differences and the often very real material barriers they raise need to be acknowledged and require complex solutions beyond what any one conference can generate.

The amendment, proposed by pro-life representatives from both parties (Stupak a Democrat and Pitts a Republican), made abortion a central sticking point of debate on the ACA. The amendment banned use of federal dollars for abortion by requiring insurers who would offer a health plan in the health exchange that included abortion to offer an identical plan without coverage and ensure that insurers used separate money for administration of the two plans. Also, anyone who received a federal subsidy for healthcare could not purchase a plan that included abortion coverage. For abortion coverage, a separate "abortion rider" would need to be purchased. Reproductive health, rights, and justice advocates opposed the amendment on many grounds.[28] First, they argued, it was redundant with the Hyde Amendment. Further, the cost of offering two plans would make insurers less likely to offer abortion coverage. Finally, women were unlikely to be able to predict future need for an abortion, and thus could not be sure beforehand of which plan to purchase.

On the Saturday evening of the conference, participants were provided a list of Democratic representatives with simple talking points: "Vote NO on Stupak Amendment" and "Vote NO on Motion to Recommit Anti Immigrant Amendment."[29] About two hundred people from the conference walked to the Capitol to visit the offices of their elected legislators, if available, or accompanied other groups. The preplanned lobby day scheduled for the Monday after the conference continued as well with about seventy participants who received a brief training on lobbying. In my volunteer role as note taker for a Management Circle meeting before the start of the conference, I observed some confusion about the planned lobby day, the first of its kind for SisterSong. In an interview, when I asked about the confusion, Ross explained why she felt this lobby day was essential: "What's the point of bringing three to four hundred women of color to Washington, DC, if we're not going to have an impact on policy? We can be meeting in Tempe, Arizona, for all it matters if you're not gonna do something on Capitol Hill."[30] The "something" had shifted in light of Saturday night's impromptu lobbying. As she was highlighting, location matters to a degree. Some places are symbolically significant whereas others are also practically significant, offering people unmatched opportunities to engage in the formal political process.

The script provided for Monday's lobby day used simple, direct messaging: "The Stupak-Pitts amendment will ban abortion coverage in the health care exchange" and "The Stupak-Pitts amendment represents a dramatic shift in federal abortion policy."[31] In the preparatory discussion, there was linking of issues (abortion, immigration status), but the talking points did not mention human rights specifically or anything beyond stating the view of the basic impact of the specific legislation. This is common in lobby days. Even though lobby days are prearranged by organizations or coalitions, legislators still have limited time to talk with constituents, and it is possible that a different issue will arise that requires cutting the meeting short or canceling it altogether. Therefore, organized lobby days aim to show that voters (or potential voters) care enough about the issue to show up in person, give a human face to the issue under discussion, and provide a unified, easily understood message—all within a matter of minutes. Thus, SisterSong's first lobby day reaffirmed Karin's point about pragmatism influencing framing. The amendment passed.[32]

A subset of interviewees who offered an important perspective were the skeptics who questioned the utility of "human rights" at a basic level. They offered a compelling logic, for different reasons, about why human rights was not a useful framing. Some, such as Sonya, a Latina Sister-Song founder who had focused on creating culturally relevant programs at Planned Parenthood, noted the explicit "academic," distancing feel of human rights discourse. Below I highlight a different reason for skepticism that an organization leader offered and place it in conversation with a SisterSong staff member. Note that while they were not literally in conversation, the juxtaposition is fruitful.

One SisterSong staff person noted that organizations had different definitions of "reproductive justice" and different relationships to human rights. She commented on the approach of a nearby organization:

> SPARK [Reproductive Justice Now! of Atlanta, Georgia], for example, doesn't really employ the human rights framework in it. We disagree with that at SisterSong. The human rights is all up and down the wall. It's written all over the wall. But SPARK doesn't really, they don't recognize a deep correlation between human rights and RJ. And so, again, everybody has a different definition. You know, a lot of us have shared definitions, yes, but there are also organizations that don't. They have created their own definition for it. It's not a bad thing. It's not a bad thing. I mean there's probably no sense to really corral everybody into one big group. But I think it is important for people to understand the human rights framework that's, the backbone of it [reproductive justice] certainly. I understand it. I understand the relevance of it.[33]

She understood that SMOs had different ideas and claimed that that was okay. Yet she also intimated that SMOs that did not use this framing did so due to a lack of understanding even though the connection to human rights was obvious ("up and down the wall" as in "the writing's on the wall"). Yet, I want to reiterate that the handful of interviewees in my study who were the most vocal critics of human rights, whom I identify as skeptics, seemed quite knowledgeable. They just did not believe in the power of a human rights frame that many scholars and activists insist exists.

For example, one interviewee questioned the strength of the idea of human rights when the political climate revealed that there were active opponents to the idea that at a basic level, everyone *is* human. I interviewed Paris Hatcher, then the co–executive director of SPARK Reproductive Justice Now! On human rights, she reflected,

So I think this is someplace where that, I know that I and also SPARK, we are divergent from like, some other organizations. Because the, the human rights piece doesn't really fit in. And I think a big piece for me is that, I mean perhaps it's that it's like, it's supposed to be sanctioned by like this UN, this other body. But we live in a culture that so much like does everything to dehumanize and uses language like "illegal alien." . . . *Because there's something about a right that just isn't powerful enough. Like it's not, those to me aren't enough, like I'm a human being so I deserve this. It doesn't resonate. You know, 'cause some people, I mean implicit in that is having people to understand that they understand their and your humanity.*[34]

On one hand, Paris questioned rights in general. On the other hand, the reason she questioned rights was her observation that rights cannot in and of themselves force people to respect one another. Astutely, this is an observation both activists and scholars alike make about rights generally, not just human rights.

When I asked more explicitly about diverging from other organizational approaches, she replied,

Yeah, yeah, because I think, like SisterSong, in example, they really undergird their work in a human rights language, and we don't. I feel like we undergird our work like in a social justice, in a social justice politic that doesn't base our deserving of, our deserving of things that we need based on our rights or someone saying that we're human, but just because that's what we, it's a fact. . . . Because I think for so many examples, like obviously when somebody puts up a billboard that says, "Black Children are an Endangered Species," it's already implicit that they don't think of us as humans. You know, like that's already there. So, to logic back that "we are human beings" doesn't work, in my opinion, 'cause they don't see it.[35]

Hatcher was referring to the 2010 Endangered Species billboard campaign that pro-life organizations developed and started in Atlanta and then spread throughout the United States. Various local organizations opposed the billboards in Atlanta, including a coalition that included SisterSong and SPARK. The controversy received national and international coverage by news media.[36] Paris's response pointed to the idea that "rights for humans" was insufficient because various people did not believe that everyone was human, so human rights advocacy was actually a nonstarter.

Paris's response surprised me for two reasons. First, what she said clearly showed skepticism—and outright rejection—of human rights, which SisterSong publicly identified as central to the framing under which the two entities regularly worked: reproductive justice. Theoretically, as a condition of joining the SisterSong coalition, organizational members such as SPARK agreed to SisterSong's Mission and Principles of Unity, which included human rights. In practice, however, there was no official process that required them to agree with every aspect. Second, the office in which I interviewed Paris had copies of the UDHR booklets, much like the ones RJ 101 workshop attendees received, resting on the board behind her. So, Paris's comments seemed to contradict this visible display of interest in human rights. But when I returned to the SPARK office to conduct a different interview, I learned that that office belonged to a different person, Tonya, a southern African American activist who had been introduced to human rights through her advocacy work in South America. Based on my interview with Tonya, she clearly felt human rights framing was a useful tool and achievement of human right a necessary goal. We can see that there are different viewpoints held within any organization or coalition, even as members work toward a common vision.

I conducted my interview with New Orleans–based organizer Shana Griffin at Hampshire College. We took a break during the Hampshire College conference referred to in the movement as "CLPP," the shortened name for the Civil Liberties and Public Policy Institute that hosted the annual event. She was an invited speaker, I an attendee. Her child played on her lap as we talked in an empty room. She reflected, "Well, I appreciate the human rights framework; I have critiques for it. But I also recognize that you have to be careful when you organize marginalized communities when you're using the framework because then people take that in and say, 'Well I have the right to this and this and this.' Human rights, as framework is important, but in terms of actual recognized rights in this country, don't exist. So it could be a set up? Yeah, it could totally be a set up." Shana's skepticism about human rights was grounded in a nuanced understanding of the relationship between the US government and the international arena. Shana expressed concern that people would want to take advantage of these rights, when they were not fully supported in the United States. She worried about human rights advocacy in the United States unintentionally creating a "set up" that misleads people: encouraging people to demand human rights when those rights were not supported through government policy.

Shana continued to reflect on why this situation existed. She noted that "the ways in which those treaties that they have signed on to, how are they implemented through current or already existing laws, it's a whole other different story. Like in this country, we sign off on all kind of stuff, but we also undermine the things on what we sign off, we put these, what they call reservations or things on them, or what have you." Here Shana was pointing to how the US government restricts human rights by signing treaties that could expand rights while simultaneously attaching reservations or limits to them. Again, as Ignatieff and others have discussed, the United States is not the only government to do this, but the United States does it at a level that few other countries can claim. Even as Shana hedged in some of her answer, she provided an incisive analysis of the relationship between international human rights and the US legal system. She continued to discuss how the United States' federated structure posed a challenge for activists seeking change and speculated about future legislation:

> The people who are using the framework have to be very conscious of how federal policies are shifting to the state level. Because a lot of things are doing this thing called devolution, where a lot of things are moving from the federal level to the state level, and when you move from the federal level to the state, you create no federal standards. If you're used to organizing from a human rights framework, that framework has no meaning without a federal standard. And no international treaty takes standard over federal law, like it has to be federally recognized, right?

Shana was clearly aware of the implications of the US government's federated structure and that, for the US government, its own laws supersede international law. Her continued discussion about the role of states in

supporting rights focused on how different social groups fared depending upon that state's history:

> And different states prioritize different resources and different communi-
> ties. So like in Louisiana, you can get welfare for two hundred dollars for
> two kids, but in places like California or Washington it's much higher.
> So we know what that looks like for people who live in the South. It's
> dominated by people who are Republican and using a neoliberal agenda.
> So, everybody can't live in a Massachusetts. . . . So, yeah, I just think it's
> important to think about how disparities and access on the state level,
> and how it's very important to fight against that. To fight for the federal
> government to always have a federal standard. Like Obama, he's done it
> with education, and even with healthcare, but they've said it's just up to
> the state, you know? They said, you know if you guys want to have this
> then it's cool, or if you don't. But that's not fair to the citizenry, because
> if you live in this state then you get fucked, and everybody will want to
> move to the other state. People are less likely to do that, but it's going to
> change if there's this influx of dark bodies, right? Poor bodies . . .

Without federal insistence on human rights, states get to choose their
approach. By states being able to choose their approach to issues
such as healthcare, citizens (and noncitizens) must rely on the moral
compass of that state's politicians, who determine budgets. As Shana
pointed out, a state's specific history, including its racial politics, influences legislators' approach to social services and rights granting. If a
state government is generous, that is beneficial, but if not, citizens are
"fucked." She was also pointing to the ways that leaders who appear
politically progressive in some instances (e.g., President Obama)
can still engage in restrictive domestication by placing responsibility
on states, which allows for decoupling of rights. Shana's views were
shaped by being based in the South and by her extensive community organizing in New Orleans and nationally with organizations
like Incite! Women of Color Against Violence. While many scholars
and activists point to the South's obvious racial history and discrimination (e.g., slavery, Jim Crow), countless studies document racial
exclusion and discriminatory policies throughout the United States.
Predictably, a specific state's "generosity" in providing social services

shifts when more racial minorities are present or perceived to be shifting the demographics.[37] Whereas Karin's reflection made clear that she thought framing issues in terms of human rights with legislators felt impractical, others such as Paris and Shana expressed concerns about audiences misunderstanding human rights or overestimating levels of government support for them.

Reworking Human Rights in the Mission

Despite these challenges, SisterSong continued to integrate human rights. In this final section, I examine the changing "place" of human rights in SisterSong by analyzing how the phrase literally moved within SisterSong's mission statement. As Blee reminds us, for movements, "Defining a problem for themselves and framing issues for external audiences are very different processes."[38] SisterSong's sixteen founding organizations developed a unified mission statement and Principles of Unity for the collective. While mission statements are usually brief, they often take time to develop since each word matters. Internally, mission statements represent ideals of what an organization is and does. Externally, mission statements are a quick way for audiences to understand the organization. While I do not discuss all the statements at length, the table summarizes some key features throughout the decades of revisions.

As previously discussed, the 1999 statement totaled three sentences:

> The SisterSong Women of Color Reproductive Health Collective is made up of local, regional and national grassroots organizations representing four primary ethnic populations/indigenous nations in the United States: Native American/Indigenous, Black/African American, Latina/ Puerto Rican and Asian/Pacific Islander. The Collective was formed with the shared recognition that as women of color we have the right and responsibility to represent ourselves and our communities. SisterSong is committed to educat[ing] women of color on Reproductive and Sexual Health and Rights and work[ing] towards the access of health services, information and resources that are culturally and linguistically appropriate through the *integration of the disciplines of community organizing, Self-Help and human rights education.*[39]

TABLE 8.1. Mission Statement Key Phrases

Year	Word count	"community organization"	"self-help"	"human rights"	HR context
1999	109	1	1	1	"HR education"; last sentence
2000	213	1	1	1	"HR advocacy"; last sentence
2002	108	1	1	1	"HR education"; last sentence
2004	115	1	1	1	"HR education"; last sentence
2005	142	1	1	2	"securing HR"; first sentence; "HR education"; last sentence
2007	142	1	1	2	"securing HR"; first sentence; "HR education"; last sentence
2016	29	0	0	1	"securing HR" (mission statement was one sentence)

The mission emphasized the importance of self-representation as both a right and a responsibility. This last sentence persisted through various revisions. In the November 2005 iteration, over a decade after SisterSong's founding, there was a small but major shift in the ordering, with human rights moving to the first sentence. The text began, "The mission of SisterSong is to amplify and strengthen the collective voices of Indigenous women and women of color *to ensure reproductive justice through securing human rights*."[40] A mission provides a vision, and in this case, securing human rights is the vision towards which to strive, whatever that means for participants. "Human rights" bookended the mission, providing a container for the rest of the work. "Human rights" was referred to variously as a strategy in service of reproductive justice and as a goal. Mission statements are idealizations, so this is the ideal vision of human rights' role even if the practice does not meet this ideal.

In 2016, almost two decades after its founding, SisterSong returned to a simple statement: "SisterSong's mission is to strengthen and amplify the collective voices of indigenous women and women of color to achieve reproductive justice by eradicating reproductive oppression and securing human rights."[41] The twenty-nine-word sentence contained elements from mission statements throughout the decades, including "collective voices." The addition of "reproductive oppression" reflected changing language in the broader movement. Even as other longstanding ideas were removed (e.g., "self-help"), "human rights" remained, demonstrating its importance to SisterSong even as the social movement sector and larger national political landscape changed. As I discuss in the conclusion, the current wave of protests suggests that an audience receptive to a human rights frame may be larger than previously envisioned. One way or another, progressives are demanding change, with the efforts of women of color being recognized in ways that they had not been previously.

Conclusion

Making Utopias Real

My book highlights the US government's engagement in restrictive domestication with which SisterSong, a leading reproductive justice organization, had to contend as its leaders engaged in revolutionary domestication to create a human rights culture. Cold War politics kept early racial justice organizations from being able to embrace human rights discourse. So, I began by asking, why would a contemporary movement choose human rights? And what does it look like to choose human rights?

In the early days, some SisterSong founders used creation of a human rights culture as a primary motivation for developing the reproductive justice framework and sought to instill this motivation in other people and continue to do so. Some of the people most committed to the idea of human rights as motivation were involved in international conferences that provided an embodied experience of connection with international women's movement activists mobilizing using the human rights framework. For other founders, this was not the case, and human rights advocacy served as more of a strategy for understanding the potential of reproductive justice to connect movements. Almost two decades after SisterSong's founding, with the mission down to one sentence, "human rights" remained: "Sister-Song's mission is to strengthen and amplify the collective voices of Indigenous women and women of color *to achieve reproductive justice by eradicating reproductive oppression and securing human rights.*"[1] Thus, irrespective of why SisterSong chose the human rights frame initially—despite changes in leadership, composition of the Management Circles, and organizational structure—human rights advocacy remains a part of SisterSong's vision.

Organizations comprise movements, and while they may enter coalition with each other at key moments, they have their own missions.

Further, individuals comprise organizations and they have their own theories of change. Rare is the organization, coalition, or movement where there is total consensus. Yet, as we see in this case, progress is possible without complete consensus. Crucially, founders agreed on the importance of understanding identities and power structures as complex and intersecting and the basis for action. Further, they agreed on the goal of organizing women of color around reproductive issues using culturally relevant approaches. Finally, they agreed on the need to change the discussion around reproduction among activists, so they would understand that reproductive rights meant little in a practical sense if women did not have the resources (economically, socially, politically) to exercise those rights, hence embracing a new language: "reproductive justice."

Of course, human rights are not a panacea and movements should not ignore multiple realities such as how key human rights documents were created with a heavy hand of Western powers that supported subordination of colonies and "third world" nations that, in turn, demanded liberation from exploitative relationships. Nor should movements ignore how nations violating human rights are simultaneously responsible for monitoring the adherence to them by other nation. Many scholars and activists who oppose human rights discourse do so on the grounds of how largely White, middle-class activists have made the claim, from a paternalistic position that works to distance oneself from being implicated in the problem of the "other." In this formulation, "they" need human rights from "us" White people because they do not understand how to operate in the world as we do. A more appealing approach for people of color is, we all need human rights because we are equally human and until you have yours, mine do not mean as much because they come at the expense of yours. Still, people can demand human rights as part of a larger vision of liberation because "rights claims are the tool, not the end of social and political struggle. It [considering the objective of the claim] nevertheless gives us a way of understanding which social movement claims for rights (amongst the present cacophony of such claims) could be considered 'progressive' because demands that seek to replace one form of power with another are not compatible with this objective of 'whittling down' the capacity of concentrated sites of power."[2] Consolidation of power is a particular concern for feminists as these institutions, whether domestic or international, rest on patriarchal foundations. Thus, "Whether one is dealing with the state, the Mafia, parents, pimps, police, or husbands, the heavy, dual price of institutionalized protection is always a measure of dependence and agreement to abide by the protector's rules."[3] The work of organizing to create a human rights culture not only asks the government to create the conditions of human thriving but also pushes the public to understand themselves as deserving of these conditions *and* as having a role in maintaining human rights through respecting each other's human rights.

Some theorists propose that we are in an era of the Anthropocene, in which human actions are destroying the planet, and thus the solution is to decenter humans and the idea of human superiority over nature in favor of a relational ontology that places humans, objects, and nature on an equal basis.[4] Yet many of these theorists inhabit bodies and positions that compose the standard image of "human" against which other groups are measured: White, English-speaking, educated, and largely male. They are neither historically nor presently in danger of treatment as anything but superior among humans. The insistence that "humans" have created these conditions conveniently places all people in the position of equally participating. Previous claims in this vein have been used to justify curtailing a range of human activity—including reproduction, which, as discussed earlier in the book, historically communities of color have disproportionately been affected by. Further, claims of rampant human destruction ignore documented caring relationships between humans and nature. For example, many Indigenous groups view humans as part of the varying components of nature, serving as current caretakers of the land. As Métis feminist anthropologist Zoe Todd notes, the insistence on moving past "the human" fails to acknowledge that insistence on human superiority has been a European and White ideology that has been perpetuated globally.[5] Thus, she encourages scholars to understand that "'Ontology' Is Just Another Word for Colonialism."[6] One prominent humanist challenges his colleagues to reject color-blind ideology that tinges the insistence on universalism and instead directly address the problems wrought through socially constructed categories such as race.[7] A criticism of human rights that undergirded my interviewee Paris's observations was noting that in a system where being human is the basis of recognition, opposing movement actors could not envision Black women's bodies *as* belonging to humans in and of themselves. Rather, Black women were receptacles for *potential* human life. Her point was that human rights advocacy was not enough because some people did not consider Black women human; before doing away with the supposed centering of humans, there is a need to cross a threshold where groups are viewed *as* human.

My initial impulse with the book title was to include the phrase "the last utopia," a concept that emerged in one historian's conclusions regarding human rights as an ideology. I agreed with his skepticism about contemporary scholars' views of the human rights concept as a panacea. Yet I also saw how people at SisterSong expressed a sense of recognition—an "aha"—when the idea was referenced. I agree with Anderson that "human rights" is specifically powerful for people inspired by the US civil rights movement, which held the attention of people beyond the United States. The phrase and the image of a world where human rights flourish hold a power whether or not academics want to believe that they should. The seeming impossibility of achieving human rights may discourage some activists from embracing them, but the very expansiveness of the framework is what draws others to it. As cultural critic Hua notes, "The conceptual conditions tied to universality, which define it through and against difference, are important to understand because they ultimately constrict how human rights can be used as a political tool even as these conditions also provide the reason why human rights offers almost limitless possibilities for imagining alternatives."[8] Imagining alternatives and trying to generate them is exactly what activists building futures seek as a long-term strategy. Thus, Crenshaw's words about how "intersectionality" has been used beyond her initial intention seem relevant here: "The point isn't to abandon the ground—the point is to battle to define what the ground means."[9] "Battleground" seems an apt description of contemporary politics, and human rights can be one tool.

Present Political Moment

In an article written over twenty years ago, Dutt concluded that the women of color who had attended UN meetings of that time felt hopeful about human rights: "This sense of affirmation had greater resonance, because of the sense of siege that pervades the political environment in the United States."[10] Since then, the US political environment has consistently produced a sense of siege among people of color in many ways. Events ranging from the Afghanistan and Iraq wars and the September 11 terrorist attacks to the election of the first Black president to the rise of the Tea Party to the economic downturn of 2008 have drastically changed the terrain in which movements engage. Politically, we are at a moment when there is a clear dissolution of the welfare state. Histories of medical abuse continue to affect women's decisions around reproductive care, and even attacks on contraception and abortion are as strong as ever.[11] I would argue, however, that context makes it even more noteworthy that SisterSong adopted such a seemingly risky approach, that of using a human rights framework. Some would argue that the vision early reproductive justice activists sought to bring forth is perhaps even farther away because of various political shifts. The 2016 election of Donald Trump demonstrates the stakes in social movements working to shift the United States to a human rights culture: the belief that we are all human is not an assumption held by all.

Governments' resistance to participation in human rights efforts is, in a way, logical. Numerous studies show that a government ratifying a human rights treaty—even without the intention of enforcing it or the resources to do so—affects that government's practices toward less repression, for example.[12] Thus, politicians who claim that even surface participation in these treaty processes or other aspects of the international human rights regime legitimate human rights are correct. As many of those politicians benefit from unequal systems, there is less motivation to change the system significantly. Participation leads to change (and some research shows that even nonparticipating countries are affected by the processes). Restrictive domestication is one of greatest discursive moves by the US government: convincing its people they already enjoy human rights, but should allow the government to spend money to "give" human rights through war and other mechanisms of violence that place human rights in jeopardy. Unless the government changes significantly by embracing a range of human rights, social movements will continue to need to engage in domestication strategies for concepts related to more radical ideas.

The US government continues to have disproportionate power in the international arena. For example, while activists have made great strides in getting governments to acknowledge sexual violence as an issue, the US government has the power to derail that progress, as demonstrated by Trump's delaying to sign a UN resolution regarding rape in conflict zones. A newspaper article observed how other governments responded: "France and Belgium also expressed disappointment at the watered down text. French permanent representative to the UN Francois Delattre said: 'We are dismayed by the fact that one state has demanded the removal of the reference to sexual and reproductive health . . . going against 25 years of gains for women's rights in situations of armed conflict.'"[13] Showing the interconnection between issues, the article noted that "in recent months, the Trump administration has taken a hard line, refusing to agree to any UN documents that refer to sexual or reproductive health, on grounds that such language implies support for abortions. It has also opposed the use of the word 'gender,' seeing it as a cover for liberal promotion of transgender rights."[14] That conservatives see reproductive autonomy, gender liberation, and human rights as connected suggests what progressive activists need to do to change the tide of US politics—"connect the dots" and forge ahead on the ground that is human rights.

A human rights frame will continue to seem novel precisely because it is downplayed in the US context. Thus, while "seeking longer-term change in hegemonic ideas is radical, and while it may decrease effectiveness in the short term or in relation to the formal political institutions of the state, it may be the only route to cultural transformations that delegitimate existing power relations."[15] Utopias offer a space for creative imagining of other possibilities. Toward the end of my second interview with Ross, we discussed how people in other countries used the phrase "reproductive justice" and whether receptivity to it emanated from its association with women of color as opposed to White, middle-class women. Ross understood the appeal as resulting from both neo-colonialism and the identity of the message's "sponsor": "Well, that's because any time you have human rights conversations, it's always initiated by those whose human rights are most violated. It's very rarely the people in power [who] initiate conversations about human rights 'cause they are not feeling the pinch or they are benefiting from the violation."[16] The tide may have turned.

The current wave of protest points to the recognition of a wider set of the population questioning the terms under which the United States is organized economically, politically, and socially. It has come after White women continued their trend of voting for Republican candidates, thereby being a key demographic to help elect Trump to office.[17] Thus, ironically, White women have mobilized in protest of other White women's (political) actions that have disproportionately affected communities of color. The Women's Marches that surprised many scholars and onlookers were preceded by years of protest by activists with Black Lives Matter, Standing Rock, and countless other demonstrations. The Women's Marches and the "pink wave" of the 2018 midterm elections point to how a wider swathe of White women are paying attention to social conditions. While SisterSong is not the entirety of the RJ movement, which continues to grow and face internal movement struggles, it remains relevant and visible on the national stage. SisterSong's current national coordinator, Monica Simpson, spoke at the 2017 DC Women's March. SisterSong was also one of the three women of color organizations that received part of the proceeds from *Together We Rise*, the official book that commemorated the 2017 marches.[18] There are new groups popping up claiming to work for justice in arenas where people of color, and particularly women of color, have been working for decades, including SisterSong. This suggests a shift in the movement sector.

SisterSong has, like other organization such as Forward Together, considered how to infuse the cultural work of artists into its campaigns—recent conferences have featured artists' images on conference material. The 2017 conference managed to be a multiracial festive event celebrating the twentieth anniversary in New Orleans. Thus, despite a hurricane bearing down on the New Orleans area that led many registered attendees to leave early or cancel coming altogether, SisterSong's energy persisted and one plenary, facilitated by my previously quoted interviewee Aimee Thorne-Thomsen, asked panelists an array of questions, including how human rights related to their work. The Black Mamas Matter Alliance that SisterSong began in 2013 continues to grow, three official Black Maternal Health Weeks have received national coverage, in 2018, 2019, and 2020, and the Black Mamas Matter Alliance is "joining dozens of global organizations who are fighting to end maternal mortality globally in advocating that the United Nations recognize April 11th as the International Day for Maternal Health and Rights."[19]

Predictably, abortion continues to take up a lot of space in the reproductive movement arena. Pew data shows that US support for abortion remains consistent: the majority favor legal abortion, though differences emerge by political party.[20] Democrats largely favor legal abortion while Republicans largely oppose it. Further, more states have proposed abortion restrictions. As of this writing, SisterSong was the lead plaintiff in a lawsuit against Georgia's Governor Kemp, who secured a contested win against Stacey Abrams in the 2018 midterm elections. *SisterSong v. Kemp* was momentous both because it was the first lawsuit in which SisterSong served as lead plaintiff and because the case was about abortion, which is not the focus of SisterSong's work historically.[21] The filing received local media attention and even *USA Today*, one of the largest US newspapers, covered the story.[22] In a press release, SisterSong's executive director, Monica Simpson, focused on the context in which people make decisions about abortion, an emphasis SisterSong took when fighting claims of "abortion as genocide" a decade prior.[23] Simpson explained SisterSong's logic in filing the lawsuit: "As a reproductive justice organization based in Georgia for over twenty years, SisterSong is committed to centering and amplifying the needs of those communities historically pushed to the margins. Georgia's maternal mortality rate is the second highest in the nation and Black women in our state are dying at six times the national average. SisterSong is bringing this lawsuit to protect maternal health and reproductive rights so that every person—especially persons of color—can thrive in their families and communities as well as *maintain their human right to make their own decisions about their reproductive lives.*"[24] In the precious space of a press release, human rights still figured prominently. These issues connected to a larger vision of thriving. The text of the case itself included reference to human rights: "By asserting the human right to reproductive justice, SisterSong works to build an effective network of individuals and organizations addressing institutional policies, systems, and cultural practices that limit the reproductive lives of marginalized people."[25] Thus the suit represented a response about abortion restrictions specifically while implying that human rights were the underlying concern for this lawsuit and would allow for the building of a network to address the myriad aspects of US society that operate through restrictive domestication. Thus, as I have shown in prior chapters, for SisterSong, the concept of human rights serves as *both* motivation and strategy. While "human rights" brings many tensions with it, it still serves as an inspiring vision.

People interested in empowering marginalized groups, without a different model of relating, will reproduce the same logics that founded the nation and the same logics of individual rights, which produce atomized spaces. The human rights framework offers a different model that, depending upon the organizing strategy, can push everyone to reconsider what they need for human flourishing *and* how they can contribute to someone else's human rights. It recalls the need to remember the words of Lilla Watson, Aboriginal activist: "If you have come to help me, you are wasting your time. But if you have come because your liberation is bound up with mine, then let us work together." This is simultaneously an old and a new movement vision as a talk one brisk night on my campus highlighted. Ericka Huggins, former Black Panther Party leader, spoke on identity, activism, and social change. As she told the audience her story of finding meditation during incarceration, dealing with the trauma of the death of her husband and fellow Party members, and seeking new ways of life, she told a story of working with children on a garden project. One boy explained to her that butterflies do not just change; they transform. She related this to broader social structures, positing that for current US society, "A change would be civil rights, which are the rights you are due by law . . . [H]uman rights, if they're honored, would be the rights you are due by your very birth. That is transformation."[26] And that transformation would be revolutionary.

ACKNOWLEDGMENTS

Now that this first book is done, my thanks are sooooo many. I will start with my family: sisters Lina and Joanne, cousin Sophie, and, of course, my mom, Toya. Genevieve, Valerie, and the Caseys as well. Mari Rodriguez Ragsdale for the reminders about the importance of ancestry. And for the love from afar, the Lunas: Carlos, Luis, and the other Colombianos.

My mom died a couple of months after I signed my book contract. But to be clear, my mother is all over this book and my work in general. In my dissertation, I thanked my mom for getting us the coolest babysitters. That was a reference to the fact that Angela Davis was babysitting my older sister when my mom went out dancing with a friend and met my dad. My mother was politically active—and balanced that with pragmatism and zest that later in life I appreciate even more. We attended the Empowering Women of Color conference at UC–Berkeley when Yuri Kochiyama spoke as the keynote. In a breakout session that I attended with my mom, she asked a question drawing on her twenty or so years of political action and working at institutions of higher education: why, twenty years later, were women of color dealing with the same problems? Today, her question is sadly still relevant, and the closer I came to finishing the book, the more I realized that while my data offers a snapshot of a time, my analysis remained relevant because social change is a long process.

Funding for the early phase of work on this book came from several grants, including the National Science Foundation Law and Social Science (#SES-0850655) and the following University of Michigan sources: the Alliance for Graduate Education and Professoriate (AGEP), the Center for Education of Women, the Department of Sociology, the Institute for Research on Women and Gender, the Nonprofit and Public Management Center, and Rackham Graduate School. I could not have written the book if the Sophia Smith Collection had not held the archival files (or if many librarians had not helped me understand unprocessed files), and of course, if SisterSong staff, movement leaders, and other activists had not agreed to interviews. Loretta Ross is hard to describe in her brilliance and charisma. While we do not always agree, she always pushes me to think.

Fellowships from the following entities provided time to write and interesting conversations: the Center for Research on Gender and Women at the University of Wisconsin–Madison's Mellon Sawyer Seminar on Globalization and the New Politics of Women's Rights; the UC President's Postdoctoral Program at UC–Berkeley, where my sponsors were Kristin Luker (Jurisprudence and Social Policy, and Sociology) and Charis Thompson (Gender and Women's Studies); and a Woodrow Wilson Career Enhancement Fellowship, during which time I was sponsored by Dorothy Roberts. At UC–Santa Barbara, a Faculty Career Development Award provided release time.

My NYU Press editor, Ilene Kalish, was funny and scary but in retrospect only in that way that New Yorkers/New Jerseyans are to the rest of the world. And she did not bat an electronic eye when I requested various changes to my contract, particularly the note about what to do in case I died during production. She just replied, "Please don't die." At an American Sociological Association meeting, we talked about writing, and she reminded me how women often feel so self-conscious about their writing, assuring me that the book did not need to be perfect and that she wanted to publish it. I said something about mentoring younger scholars. She stopped with the smiles, looked at me directly, and said plainly, "Mentor yourself." Hers is an important message for all, especially women of color. It is a testament to Ilene's feminist praxis that her catalogue is a daring, diverse one. Across several sets of reviewers' comments, I felt how people were taking my work seriously and wanted to fully develop its potential to have the widest influence—thank you for the thoughtful, compassionate critique. Assistant Editor Sonia Tsuruoka enthusiastically answered my many questions. I am honored to be part of the NYU Press family.

Writing can be a lonely process, but my working groups have been a key sounding board. For over fifteen years, G3SG has met biweekly in person or virtually. Laura Hirshfield, Emily Kazyak, Carla Pfeffer, and K. Scherrer—thank you for so many conversations, laughs, and recipes. It is hard to put into words what you have meant as scholars and friends. It would take a whole other book. To Katherine Luke—while you have done many awesome things, including having two sweet kids, I am forever grateful that you included me in that initial e-mail inquiry about forming a group. We miss you and know you would be so proud of the community we have built.

The Writing Group has remained a source of support from those initial days meeting in the downstairs of the Michigan Union over a decade ago. Our current configuration of Kristen Hopewell, Maria S. Johnson, and Lynn Verduzco-Baker has met across continents. My most recent group, the small but mighty Scholars Network for Reproductive Justice (SNRJ): Anu Gomez, Krystale Littlejohn, and LaKisha Simmons. I love creating a space with other junior(ish) scholars of color who work from a reproductive justice ethic as we grapple with the contradictions of the academy.

Write-on-sites (WOS) have been an important space for me, from the first I created in the Bay Area with other postdocs, visitors, and independent scholars. The Bay Area Write-on-Site I started included Liberty Barnes, James Battle, Anne Finger (who modestly mentioned having done some reproductive activism), Liza Fuentes, Chris Hannsmann, Tomomi Kinukawa, Sarah Lamble, Christin Munsch, Victor Pineda, and Danielle Watts. At UC–Santa Barbara, in my second quarter, I sought out a fellow NCFDD fan, Sarah Roberts, in Education. We started UCSB WOS with one Wednesday a week; then it became two days a week. Since then the WOS community expanded to seven weekly sessions hosted by different people across campus (and off campus), and writing retreats sponsored by the Office of Research (thanks, Barbara Walker).

Over the years I had many crucial conversations with people about "the book" and my goals for it: Chris N. J. Roberts, Sylvanna Falcón, Jennifer Nelson, and, at UC–Santa Barbara, Alison Brysk and my hallway neighbor, Eddie Telles, who had worked at Ford Foundation, and Lisa Hajjar. I would also like to thank people who read specific parts of the book: Beth Schneider, Verta Taylor, and Belinda Robnett all helped me craft a successful proposal. Kim Greenwell for the pushes and cheerleading. I thank the UC–Santa Barbara Health, Medicine, and Care Working Group, particularly Laury Oaks, Lisa S. Park, Barbara Herr Harthorn, and Eileen Boris for lively discussion on earlier chapters. Grace L.

Sanders and Dorothy Roberts asked key questions during my visit to Penn's Alice Paul Center for Research on Women and Gender, which helped me reshape the draft. My Santa Barbara crew helped me build a solid foundation: Sarah Roberts, Micaela-Diaz Sanchez, Stacey Beauregard, Dannah Perez, Maren Lange, and Jamie Thomas.

For physical writing space, I have benefited from generosity throughout the world. I thank Kiran Asher, whose impromptu offer after Jade Sasser's "Old Maps, New Terrain" convening made another trip to the Sophia Smith archive possible. Nupur, Virali, and little Anika Modi-Parekh, who, upon receiving my e-mail from a friend of a friend, invited me to house sit. I wrote, watered tomatoes, and reflected on community praxis. Because what better represents the type of world we want to live in than people sharing what they have with each other? After my Woodrow Wilson interview in January 2017 in Philly, I took the train to Ginger Luke and Don Chery's house in the DMV region and two days later collected data on the ground at the Women's March in DC. Nine months later their bustling house became a space from which to grieve, write, and witness that unbelievably strange yet mundane place that is our nation's capital. Being in the place where the paper reports on local news that for everyone else is national news and where sometimes you turn right instead of left at certain Metro stops and find yourself running into a monument rather than the coffee shop at which you planned to do some work and then can stop by the Supreme Court for a brief tour or watch a tax protest adds a different lens to the writing. Michelle Kuo and Albert Wu, whom I met at Michelle's open mic night in Paris on my mom's birthday. A few days later, we got drinks and swapped stories about social justice and university life. The next day, Michelle and I got to meet the esteemed Patricia J. Williams at the Quai Branley museum, and a week(ish) later I was house sitting in their flat. At Michelle and Albert's place, I was surrounded by familiar books, some of which are cited here. And I got to bake cookies in a real oven.

Myra Marx Ferree selected me for the Sawyer Seminar on Human Rights postdoctoral fellowship at UW–Madison. She is wicked smart and not afraid to be a "difficult woman" and let us know how much she expects of us. It is an honor. Jennifer Reich pulled me aside at a Sociologists for Women in Society conference to ask about the book and offered to read chapters—then actually did it and offered painstaking notes. Thanks, Kristin Luker, my UC President's Postdoc Fellowship mentor—who agreed to be my sponsor (thanks, Elena Gutiérrez for the idea) and with whom I would meet in person and virtually for years after my fellowship ended. Our friendship grew over the years. She reached out to me in summer 2018 and agreed to an emergency Skype call during which she listened with her trademark nonjudgmental soft smile. After my word vomit, she offered her analysis: "It sounds like you've lost your voice." Then she reminded me of Annie Lamott's words: perfectionism is the voice of the oppressor. After that conversation, I reread my pre-professor articles and remembered what it was like to write without having a stadium of (inner) critics surrounding me (or at least a smaller stadium). Kara Lowentheil and Krista St. James helped me work on taming those lizard-y critics, too. Dorothy Roberts, who is somehow simultaneously brilliant, gracious, funny, and prolific—words cannot describe the foundation you have built for our work and how you continue to serve as a North Star for so many of us. You continued to remind me that women of color are valuable to study in and of ourselves, even when Sociology refuses to believe so.

Over the years many undergraduates assisted me with finding an item for a footnote or reading some part of a chapter and helping me produce an accessible book that could reach a wider audience. At UC–Berkeley, many students from the Undergraduate Research Assistance Program engaged in conversations about reproductive justice and human rights: Darlene Olmedo, Elvina Fan, Emma Ireland, and Michael Traber. At UC–Santa Barbara, students in the Faculty Research Assistance Program (FRAP) offered a keen eye on different chapters and asked questions that reminded me why I wanted future generations of students to learn from my book: Angelica Quintana, Caroline Arzoo, Gabby Waltz, Jessica Lau, Kellie McManamon, Mollie Kraus, Natalia Gonzalez, Samantha Cheney, Sam Mejia, and Tom Moskowitz. Special thanks to FRAP student Farzana Rahman, who asked thoughtful questions in my Women's Movement class and applied that inquisitiveness as she read various chapter drafts, pushing the work further. She also researched some footnotes and found additional sources.

Lalaie Ameeriar, my grief buddy, who understood how the academic enterprise loses meaning when you are adjusting to life in which the only mother you have known is dead. Hahrie Han, thank you for the tea. Colleagues such as France Winddance Twine, Howie Winant, Maria Charles, Sarah Thébaud, Kum-Kum Bhavnani, and John Mohr graciously welcomed me to the department. A particular thanks to Myra Marx Ferree (again), George Lipsitz, Kristin Luker (again), Laury Oaks, Hahrie Han (again), Victor Rios (again), Leila Rupp, Verta Taylor, and Vilna Bashi Treitler for reminding me that I could write this book. And for bold movement thinkers and theorists—Roula AbiSamra, Jill Adams, Juana Rosa Cuavera, Sujatha Jesudason, Laura Jiménez, Mimi Kim, Shanelle Matthews, and Becky Smith—who in their own ways reminded me that I could benefit the movement just as I am. You continue to inspire me with your warmth, wit, and wisdom.

APPENDIX A

Methods

Over the years, my relationship to the RJ movement has shifted. Concerns about affecting the research site can be especially salient when one is studying social movements and social movement organizations because social movement participants are "in the business of trying to convince people of the wisdom or folly of a given social or personal reality."[1] However, it is important to note that in some settings, movement actors are resistant to research being conducted without tangible benefit to them, so access is not allowed *without* participation. At points in the research, movement participants (not all necessarily interviewees) made comments that suggested that my participant observation had given me sustained visibility. This increased my legitimacy as a researcher and gave me more access than I would have gained solely through conducting interviews or document analysis. I also participated in two other important activities. The first was a year-long internship in the 501 c3 Advocacy division of a Planned Parenthood office from 2008 to 2009. The second was participation in the United Nations 53rd Commission on the Status of Women in 2009 in New York. While these were not formal data-collection experiences, they provided insight into the broader field of reproductive politics and international women's advocacy.

The documents I use as data came from five sources: the Sophia Smith Collection Women's History Archive at Smith College; SisterSong's national office, where staff gave me access to the server and the file cabinets; publicly available documents on the SisterSong websites; similar documents from other reproductive justice organizations; and, finally, documents individuals gave me. Some researchers, such as Lofland, differentiate between documents available in a formal archive (archival documents) and documents produced by a movement (movement publications).[2] Other researchers, such as Yin, do not differentiate on the argument that the biases of such types of documents are similar—namely, they can be produced with a specific audience in mind, which can reflect an ideal rather than an "objective" reality.[3] Of course, feminist scholars have long noted that objectivity is a social construct. Since my initial data collection, archiving software has improved and there are services online that allow for different types of searches, such as the Internet Wayback Machine. So, I draw on official documents such as meeting minutes, newspapers, and public interviews, but also other sources of data marked "confidential," e-mails stored on servers, and revelations whispered to me in private conversation with the stated desire of inclusion in research under promise of anonymity. During participant observation, I also gathered materials (e.g., brochures, stickers, etc.) that I treated as movement artifacts rather than documents.[4] Treating them as such, I did not attempt to code them, in part because some were difficult to physically scan, such as the condoms that were often included in registration folders at SisterSong conferences. These items are indeed significant but not central to the themes explored in this book.

There are different sites of contestation, the analysis of which would allow us to examine this story in significantly different ways: a front-stage/backstage analysis comparing what is in the documents versus what is said in interviews; the different types of people involved in early days and their views on human rights—true believers/proselytizers, undecided/ambivalent, and skeptics; and, as always with movements, the dynamics of internal politics. Each approach has an advantage and disadvantage, privileging some narratives over others and therefore some voices over others. Yet in that privileging we lose some aspects of the story that would otherwise help us understand the pathways and meanings given to and by the different actors involved.

All academic work is knowledge production, which is always political. Writing about contemporary social movements is particularly complex as it involves understanding the lives of people attempting to make social change, albeit with sometimes-conflicting visions and, as interviewees shared, personalities. Those attempts can be fraught with challenges both external and internal. The internal typically poses the greatest challenge to researchers, particularly those of us with more than a passing interest in what we research. Interviewees invest a level of trust in us to tell their story, but as social scientists our task is to place that story in context and sometimes that context is not complimentary. Moreover, rarely is the situation as simple as interviewees present it because humans are, well, human and our perspective is partial.

As each year passed, I had more questions about the content and implications of my research. In the early years of my research, other academics assumed I was actively involved in RJ because I shared an identity with many of my interviewees—woman of color. I was working on data collection, sometimes teaching, and navigating the rest of my life. So, I visited the reproductive justice movement. I applied for a scholarship to attend conferences. In exchange for scholarships, recipients worked at the conferences. One time this meant I was assisting in presenting a workshop with SisterSong's communications manager. In the book's opening scene at the LTAS Miami conference, multiple attendees assumed I was going to be in the Black reproductive justice photo and reminded me when and where the photo would be taken. As with other aspects of the movement, I did not claim a "right" to be involved but if invited in, I generally went. My aim was to write a theoretically rich and methodologically rigorous study. People in the movement volunteered their hopes for my research: after I visited the SisterSong office for an RJ 101 training, Loretta Ross told me she was glad I was doing the research because women of color needed to do more theorizing. At other times people told me they understood I would not "air dirty laundry"—a promise that I did not make but that they felt was implied by a shared racial/gender identity. From the beginning of my research I was given multiple mandates by other people: as a woman of color I had something special to offer, many people intoned, and I was told I must avoid "airing dirty laundry" while at the same time I was asked to do things like take notes at a private meeting once so I would see that SisterSong was not "all peaches and cream."

I was looking through the SisterSong website one day and was surprised to find one of my articles listed as a resource. Another time I visited the site and saw I was in one of the rotating pictures. Two of us who had met with the office Michigan US Representative John Dingell stood in front of his office with the state seal behind us. The photo clearly identified us: "Seema Singh and Zakiya Luna at Dingell's office." Since some of these events predated the proliferation of social media, whatever photos we sent the staff seemed valuable. Yet, I continued to be surprised finding myself on the website.

Over the years my "visits" became longer and because I was one of the early scholars studying the movement *as* a movement, more people began to reach out to me. In early years I sent an article draft to interviewees for any feedback—none provided any although a year after its publication one reached out to congratulate me on it. People are busy!

Sometimes by pure accident I have ended up on e-mail lists with confidential conversations. At various reproductive justice events, I would interview people and then hours later they would invite me to hang out for a meal and ask my perspective on an issue in the movement or their organization. Or people would invite me to go dance—an invitation I declined as I was trying to determine the line between researcher and activist. Even after I finished the initial data collection and became more involved with the movements, people seemed to understand me as a researcher, or "professor," as some called me years later.

At UC–Berkeley, when I was a UC President's Postdoctoral Fellow, I was housed in the new Center on Reproductive Rights and Justice at Berkeley Law (CRRJ), the brainchild of noted scholars of reproduction Kristin Luker and Jill Adams, who while at Boalt Hall had taken a class from Krista. Jill went on to direct Law Students for Reproductive Choice (now If/When/How: Lawyering for Reproductive Justice). I began my postdoc a week before Jill began as CRRJ's inaugural executive director while Krista was the faculty director. CRRJ was initially an unfunded entity composed of two individual offices and a cubicle where I sat. I became what we sometimes jokingly referred to as an "accidental cofounder." Through CRRJ I learned so many things and most importantly developed loving friendships. I started the nation's first Reproductive Justice Working Group, which brought together academics and activists from throughout the Bay Area and farther reaches. Further, I coordinated the intergenerational Conversations in Reproductive Justice program, and gave feedback on the first casebook on reproductive rights law, which CRRJ produced.[5] The experience had a sense of newness and of coming full circle when CRRJ hosted Elena Gutiérrez as a visiting scholar during her sabbatical.

I still remember getting drinks at a reproductive justice social where I was reminded that people had not forgotten my role as a researcher. Someone discussed a situation between a couple of movement leaders, then turned to me and said, "Don't put that in the book," with a laugh. That story and the many others I heard over the years stayed out of this book and articles I have written. Still, they all helped me understand the complexity of the broader movement. Further, my understanding of the necessity of bringing light to movement struggles also changed over the years as it became clear that denying these realities could at times prove detrimental later. I have received both praise for documenting the history of reproductive justice and critique for some of my conclusions and have had my commitment to reproductive justice questioned. I experience a version of an outsider-within.[6] The longer my time engaging with reproductive health, rights, and justice activism (including as CoreAlign fellow and serving on the board of an RJ organization), the more complex the story, which I believe is the way it should be. Writing my first articles on reproductive justice activism, which highlighted the tensions between women of color and White women, were in retrospect easier than my later *Gender and Society* article focusing on how women of color engage in coalition politics together. While one senior scholar told me, "We don't need another piece on coalition," I knew I was onto something when I presented on the concepts at the UC–Berkeley Center for Race and Gender forum alongside Sujatha Jesudason. During Q & A, someone said of my presentation that the organization she was with had the same issues and the audience laughed and some others offered "yes." What one activist calls "dirty laundry" another activist sees as part of the conversation that allows the movement to progress rather than repeat frustrating patterns. Exchanges like these that happened far away from SisterSong's Atlanta office or events highlighted how entering and exiting the field is, in some ways, never done.

Currently in sociology, there are calls for interdisciplinary scholarship, for practical application, for scholars of movements, a connection to movements. Yet, this is also what leads to claims of bias in research. I am also sometimes skeptical of claims of scholar-activism and work "for the community" as it now appears fashionable to title everything from writing a blog post critiquing the academy to protesting in the streets as scholar activism. Women of color in the academy—and those who left the academy—have been doing this work for decades.[7] Whatever people want to call this process, I hope the ever-expanding network of reproductive justice scholars and activists finds value in the analysis I offer here.

Universal Declaration of Human Rights

PREAMBLE

Whereas recognition of the inherent dignity and of the equal and inalienable rights of all members of the human family is the foundation of freedom, justice and peace in the world,

Whereas disregard and contempt for human rights have resulted in barbarous acts which have outraged the conscience of mankind, and the advent of a world in which human beings shall enjoy freedom of speech and belief and freedom from fear and want has been proclaimed as the highest aspiration of the common people,

Whereas it is essential, if man is not to be compelled to have recourse, as a last resort, to rebellion against tyranny and oppression, that human rights should be protected by the rule of law,

Whereas it is essential to promote the development of friendly relations between nations,

Whereas the peoples of the United Nations have in the Charter reaffirmed their faith in fundamental human rights, in the dignity and worth of the human person and in the equal rights of men and women and have determined to promote social progress and better standards of life in larger freedom,

Whereas Member States have pledged themselves to achieve, in cooperation with the United Nations, the promotion of universal respect for and observance of human rights and fundamental freedoms,

Whereas a common understanding of these rights and freedoms is of the greatest importance for the full realization of this pledge,

Now, Therefore THE GENERAL ASSEMBLY proclaims THIS UNIVERSAL DECLARATION OF HUMAN RIGHTS as a common standard of achievement for all peoples and all nations, to the end that every individual and every organ of society, keeping this Declaration constantly in mind, shall strive by teaching and education to promote respect for these rights and freedoms and by progressive measures, national and international, to secure their universal and effective recognition and observance, both among the peoples of Member States themselves and among the peoples of territories under their jurisdiction.

ARTICLE 1.

All human beings are born free and equal in dignity and rights. They are endowed with reason and conscience and should act towards one another in a spirit of brotherhood.

ARTICLE 2.

Everyone is entitled to all the rights and freedoms set forth in this Declaration, without distinction of any kind, such as race, colour, sex, language, religion, political or other opinion, national or social origin, property, birth or other status. Furthermore, no distinction shall be made on the basis of the political, jurisdictional or international status of the country or territory to which a person belongs, whether it be independent, trust, non-self-governing or under any other limitation of sovereignty.

ARTICLE 3.

Everyone has the right to life, liberty and security of person.

ARTICLE 4.

No one shall be held in slavery or servitude; slavery and the slave trade shall be prohibited in all their forms.

ARTICLE 5.

No one shall be subjected to torture or to cruel, inhuman or degrading treatment or punishment.

ARTICLE 6.

Everyone has the right to recognition everywhere as a person before the law.

ARTICLE 7.

All are equal before the law and are entitled without any discrimination to equal protection of the law. All are entitled to equal protection against any discrimination in violation of this Declaration and against any incitement to such discrimination.

ARTICLE 8.
Everyone has the right to an effective remedy by the competent national tribunals for acts violating the fundamental rights granted him by the constitution or by law.

ARTICLE 9.
No one shall be subjected to arbitrary arrest, detention or exile.

ARTICLE 10.
Everyone is entitled in full equality to a fair and public hearing by an independent and impartial tribunal, in the determination of his rights and obligations and of any criminal charge against him.

ARTICLE 11.
(1) Everyone charged with a penal offence has the right to be presumed innocent until proved guilty according to law in a public trial at which he has had all the guarantees necessary for his defence.
(2) No one shall be held guilty of any penal offence on account of any act or omission which did not constitute a penal offence, under national or international law, at the time when it was committed. Nor shall a heavier penalty be imposed than the one that was applicable at the time the penal offence was committed.

ARTICLE 12.
No one shall be subjected to arbitrary interference with his privacy, family, home or correspondence, nor to attacks upon his honour and reputation. Everyone has the right to the protection of the law against such interference or attacks.

ARTICLE 13.
(1) Everyone has the right to freedom of movement and residence within the borders of each state.
(2) Everyone has the right to leave any country, including his own, and to return to his country.

ARTICLE 14.

(1) Everyone has the right to seek and to enjoy in other countries asylum from persecution.

(2) This right may not be invoked in the case of prosecutions genuinely arising from non-political crimes or from acts contrary to the purposes and principles of the United Nations.

ARTICLE 15.

(1) Everyone has the right to a nationality.

(2) No one shall be arbitrarily deprived of his nationality nor denied the right to change his nationality.

ARTICLE 16.

(1) Men and women of full age, without any limitation due to race, nationality or religion, have the right to marry and to found a family. They are entitled to equal rights as to marriage, during marriage and at its dissolution.

(2) Marriage shall be entered into only with the free and full consent of the intending spouses.

(3) The family is the natural and fundamental group unit of society and is entitled to protection by society and the State.

ARTICLE 17.

(1) Everyone has the right to own property alone as well as in association with others.

(2) No one shall be arbitrarily deprived of his property.

ARTICLE 18.

Everyone has the right to freedom of thought, conscience and religion; this right includes freedom to change his religion or belief, and freedom, either alone or in community with others and in public or private, to manifest his religion or belief in teaching, practice, worship and observance.

ARTICLE 19.

Everyone has the right to freedom of opinion and expression; this right includes freedom to hold opinions without interference and to seek, receive and impart information and ideas through any media and regardless of frontiers.

ARTICLE 20.

(1) Everyone has the right to freedom of peaceful assembly and association.

(2) No one may be compelled to belong to an association.

ARTICLE 21.

(1) Everyone has the right to take part in the government of his country, directly or through freely chosen representatives.

(2) Everyone has the right of equal access to public service in his country.

(3) The will of the people shall be the basis of the authority of government; this will shall be expressed in periodic and genuine elections which shall be by universal and equal suffrage and shall be held by secret vote or by equivalent free voting procedures.

ARTICLE 22.

Everyone, as a member of society, has the right to social security and is entitled to realization, through national effort and international cooperation and in accordance with the organization and resources of each State, of the economic, social and cultural rights indispensable for his dignity and the free development of his personality.

ARTICLE 23.

(1) Everyone has the right to work, to free choice of employment, to just and favourable conditions of work and to protection against unemployment.

(2) Everyone, without any discrimination, has the right to equal pay for equal work.

(3) Everyone who works has the right to just and favourable remuneration ensuring for himself and his family an existence worthy of human dignity, and supplemented, if necessary, by other means of social protection.

(4) Everyone has the right to form and to join trade unions for the protection of his interests.

ARTICLE 24.

Everyone has the right to rest and leisure, including reasonable limitation of working hours and periodic holidays with pay.

ARTICLE 25.

(1) Everyone has the right to a standard of living adequate for the health and well-being of himself and of his family, including food, clothing, housing and medical care and necessary social services, and the right to security in the event of unemployment, sickness, disability, widowhood, old age or other lack of livelihood in circumstances beyond his control.

(2) Motherhood and childhood are entitled to special care and assistance. All children, whether born in or out of wedlock, shall enjoy the same social protection.

ARTICLE 26.

(1) Everyone has the right to education. Education shall be free, at least in the elementary and fundamental stages. Elementary education shall be compulsory. Technical and professional education shall be made generally available and higher education shall be equally accessible to all on the basis of merit.

(2) Education shall be directed to the full development of the human personality and to the strengthening of respect for human rights and fundamental freedoms. It shall promote understanding, tolerance and friendship among all nations, racial or religious groups, and shall further the activities of the United Nations for the maintenance of peace.

(3) Parents have a prior right to choose the kind of education that shall be given to their children.

ARTICLE 27.

(1) Everyone has the right freely to participate in the cultural life of the community, to enjoy the arts and to share in scientific advancement and its benefits.

(2) Everyone has the right to the protection of the moral and material interests resulting from any scientific, literary or artistic production of which he is the author.

ARTICLE 28.

Everyone is entitled to a social and international order in which the rights and freedoms set forth in this Declaration can be fully realized.

ARTICLE 29.

(1) Everyone has duties to the community in which alone the free and full development of his personality is possible.

(2) In the exercise of his rights and freedoms, everyone shall be subject only to such limitations as are determined by law solely for the purpose of securing due recognition and respect for the rights and freedoms of others and of meeting the just requirements of morality, public order and the general welfare in a democratic society.

(3) These rights and freedoms may in no case be exercised contrary to the purposes and principles of the United Nations.

ARTICLE 30.

Nothing in this Declaration may be interpreted as implying for any State, group or person any right to engage in any activity or to perform any act aimed at the destruction of any of the rights and freedoms set forth herein.

NOTES

INTRODUCTION

1 One of my interviewees, activist Paris Hatcher, organized the "Black RJ" photo and the next one taken at the LTAS conference in 2017. The 2017 photo included men and gender- nonconforming people and is visible on SisterSong's webpage that explains the history of RJ: "About Us," SisterSong, https://www.sistersong.net. Throughout, I use the gender language taken directly from data such as documents and interviews, research articles, and the like.

2 Ross 2006, 1. SisterSong replaced "health" with "justice" in 2010.

3 SisterSong, "LR and TBL Welcome Letter." SisterSong server, July 14, 2011, in author's possession.

4 One set of people understood burlesque as an empowering form of self-expression by women of color taking control of their sexuality, whereas another set understood burlesque as like stripping/exotic dancing, which was argued to be exploitative, so they did not want SisterSong formally supporting BGB. The May prior, SisterSong's policy call for members focused on sex work. While the proposal of having a burlesque performance was the impetus for the call, the focus was beyond that, as demonstrated by panelists beyond SisterSong: Brown Girl Burlesque, Critical Resistance, and Young-Women's Empowerment Project (Y-WEP). The speakers offered different perspectives on burlesque specifically and "sex work" broadly. Y-WEP even refused the terms of engagement, noting that for their organization "sex work" was a misnomer because not all people experienced their activity as "work." Rather, some experienced it as "getting by." Further, in some cases, there was direct coercion, hence the suggestion that this was chosen "work" for those people was inaccurate. The conversations leading up to the policy call and the call itself were passionate presentations that offered extensive information and surprising personal revelations of involvement in sex work. The actual show was well attended. Since then, BGB has received national media attention—see https://browngirlsburlesque.com. For more on burlesque and debates on its relationship to feminist politics and capitalism, see Kay Siebler, "What's So Feminist about Garters and Bustiers? Neo-Burlesque as Post-Feminist Sexual Liberation," *Journal of Gender Studies* 24.5 (2015): 561–73. https://doi.org/10.10 80/09589236.2013.861345. While there are few studies on burlesque in general, one that explicitly draws attention to intersections of race, class, and disability is a recent dissertation (see Casely Emma Coan, 2019 "Kai(e)Rotic Moments:

Resistance and Alternate Futures in Burlesque Performance" (dissertation), Department of Rhetoric, Composition, and the Teaching of English, University of Arizona. https://repository.arizona.edu).

5 SisterSong mission statement. SisterSong server, 2005, emphasis added.

6 Levitsky 2007.

7 Althusser 1970; Smith 2007.

8 I thank Dorothy Roberts for initial discussion around this point.

9 A complete history is beyond the scope of the book, but has been chronicled in other places. See my other writings and Silliman et al. 2004; Price 2010; and Ross et al. 2017.

10 Ross 2006, 1.

11 Roth 2004, 3.

12 Melucci 1994; Van Dyke, Soule, and Taylor 2004.

13 Mansbridge and Morris 2001.

14 Bernstein 2005; Hunt, Benford, and Snow 1994; Polletta and Jasper 2001.

15 Taylor and Whittier 1992.

16 Some people use these terms interchangeably. It is beyond the scope of my book to address the vociferous debates about types of feminism. Still, there is a distinction between "mainstream feminism" identified in the wave analogy and what some people are now calling "intersectional feminism," which attends to intersections of race, gender, and class in their entirety, or as interlocking systems of oppression and privilege. Some books that engage these distinctions include Anzaldúa 1990; Baumgardner and Richards 2000; Heywood and Drake 1997; Labaton and Martin 2009; Walker 1995.

17 Thompson 2002, 342.

18 Inuzuka 1991, 1222.

19 Western States Center 2011.

20 Wade 2011.

21 The 1977 National Women's Conference: American Women on the Move (NWC) was held in Texas. It was an outgrowth of the UN Decade on Women (1975–1985). Presidents Ford and Carter supported the NWC. Congress funded the NWC, which would eventually produce a Plan of Action to present to Congress. Further, Congress funded pre-NWC state conventions in which attendees developed area "planks" composed of various resolutions for consideration at the NWC. At the state preconventions, delegates for the later NWC were selected. From these various conventions, twenty-six planks were produced. Before the NWC, White conference organizers such as Ellie Smeal, seemingly without consulting minority women, wrote a two-hundred-page draft document that included a three-paragraph "minority women's plank." Dissatisfied with this approach, a group of Black women produced their own Black Women's Agenda (BWA) that they aimed to have NWC delegates vote to include in the report. Women of other ethnic backgrounds developed minority-

specific caucuses at the NWC and produced agendas as well. Eventually the groups came together, generating a Minority Women's Plank that discussed issues faced by minorities writ large and concerns specific to each minority group. Sources include Cynthia Salzman Mondell and Allen Mondell, "Sisters of '77," PBS, Independent Lens, 2017, available at https://www.pbs.org; "Minority Women," Women on the Move: Texas and the Fight for Women's Rights, May 24, 2019, retrieved from https://www.womenonthemovetx.com; A. Q. Timis, "Women's Conference Approves Planks on Abortion and Rights for Homosexuals," *New York Times*, November 21, 1988, https://www.nytimes.com; Document 25, Women and Social Movements in the United States, 1600-2000, Alexander Street, https://womhist.alexanderstreet.com, accessed February 14, 2020; "The Minority Caucus: 'It's Our Movement Now,'" National Commission on the Observance of International Women's Year, *The Spirit of Houston: The First National Women's Conference* (Washington, DC: US Government Printing Office, 1978), 156–57, included in *How Did the National Women's Conference in Houston in 1977 Shape a Feminist Agenda for the Future?*—documents selected and interpreted by Kathryn Kish Sklar and Thomas Dublin with research assistance by Sandra Henderson (Binghamton, NY: State University of New York at Binghamton, 2004).

22 Cottrell 2010.

23 Steinman 2012.

24 See my previous writing on the complexity of the concept: Luna 2016.

25 The goals of these movements have not necessarily been achieved in their entirety, and some people continue to work towards those visions, but the peak time of mobilization associated with those movements has ended.

26 Okamoto 2003; Daisy Verduzco Reyes, "Inhabiting Latino Politics: How Colleges Shape Students' Political Styles," *Sociology of Education* 88.4 (2015) 302–19; Steinman 2012.

27 See *Sociological Focus* 49.1, a special issue on Black Movements edited by Joyce Bell.

28 Combahee River Collective 1983, 275.

29 Crenshaw 1989, 139; King 1988.

30 Cole and Luna 2010.

31 Rudy 2000.

32 Eschle 2002.

33 Stern 2005; Paul A. Lombardo, *Three Generations, No Imbeciles: Eugenics, the Supreme Court, and Buck V. Bell.* Baltimore, MD: John Hopkins University Press, 2008.

34 Sheba George, Nelida Duran, and Keith Norris, "A Systematic Review of Barriers and Facilitators to Minority Research Participation among African Americans, Latinos, Asian Americans, and Pacific Islanders," *American Journal of Public Health* 104.2 (2013): e16–31. Harriet A. Washington, *Medical Apartheid: The Dark*

History of Medical Experimentation on Black Americans from Colonial Times to the Present (New York: Doubleday, 2006).

35 The phrase comes from Hamer's speech at the Democratic Convention in 1963. "Fannie Lou Hamer's Speeches," Jackson State University, http://www.jsums.edu.

36 Loyd 2014.

37 Nelson 2011.

38 Nelson 2003.

39 Hertel and Libal 2011.

40 Blau et al. 2008; Hertel and Libal 2011.

41 For arguments about the timing of the Court's decision around *Roe* see Balkin 2005; Halfmann 2011; Rosenberg 1991.

42 The ruling dismissed requiring notification of spouse. At the initial time of writing, thirty-four states had a combination of counseling/waiting periods, and some require fetal imaging as part of the pre-abortion counseling. See "Counseling and Waiting Periods for Abortion," Guttmacher Institute, https://www.guttmacher.org (last accessed May 1, 2019).

43 Springer 2005.

44 Not all illegal abortions were unsafe. See Solinger 2001.

45 Other areas where this concern was reflected were artistic works such as those of noted Black feminist poet Audre Lourde.

46 Snow et al. 1986.

47 Croteau and Hicks 2003.

48 Carragee and Roefs 2004.

49 Steinberg 1999, 742.

50 Ferree 2003.

51 M. W. Steinberg, "The Talk and Back Talk of Collective Action: A Dialogic Analysis of Repertoires of Discourse among Nineteenth-Century English Cotton Spinners," *American Journal of Sociology* 105.3 (1999).

52 M. W. Steinberg, "The Talk and Back Talk of Collective Action: A Dialogic Analysis of Repertoires of Discourse among Nineteenth-Century English Cotton Spinners," *American Journal of Sociology* 105.3 (1999): 742.

53 Horton 2010; Reese and Newcombe 2003.

54 Ferree et al. 2002.

55 Ferree 2003, 339.

56 Soohoo 2008; Bernstein and Naples 2015. There are also theories about global diffusion of norms, but those are not my focus.

57 Merry 2006.

58 Levitt and Merry 2009, 457–58.

59 Levitt and Merry 2009, 443.

60 Merry et al. 2010; Rosen and Yoon 2009.

61 Finnegan, Saltsman, and White 2010; Landy 2013.

62 Pearce 2001.

63 Somers and Roberts 2008.

64 Sjoberg, Gill, and Williams 2001.

65 Armaline, Glasberg, and Purkayastha 2017, 222.

66 Brunsma, Smith, and Gran 2015.

67 Clément 2015, 564.

68 Blau 2017, 226, emphasis added.

69 I also worked as a research assistant on the larger project from 2006 to 2009. My assignments included researching footnotes to clarify terms. The project expanded to include other countries beyond the original four. Free transcripts, video, and teaching materials are available at "Resources," Global Feminisms Project, https://globalfeminisms.umich.edu.

70 Yin 2003, 93.

71 Emerson, Fretz, and Shaw 1995; Lofland 1996; Lofland et al. 2006.

72 Collins and Bilge 2016.

73 Choo and Ferree 2010.

74 Thompson 2002.

CHAPTER 1. RESTRICTIVE DOMESTICATION

1 See Anderson 2003.

2 Moyn 2010b, 9.

3 For texts that delve further into this topic, see Bogost 2012.

4 See appendix B for the text of the UDHR.

5 Donnelly 2007, 5.

6 Some scholars note that while historically we can find allusions to morality across many societies, "it has been the influence of the West, including the Western conception of universal rights, that has prevailed." Ishay 2008, 7. In critiquing what he describes as Critical Race and LatCrit theorists' simplistic embrace of international human rights law, Eric Heinz writes, "An internationalist fairyland may indeed tell us that the UN emerged out of 'vastly different ideological views.' But history recites a rather bleaker tale. The idea of an overarching system of international law replete with a 'United Nations,' and a sufficiently shared set of norms and concepts, surfaces only at that moment in world history when sufficient human diversity has been either exterminated or subordinated by big powers." More recently, Moyn has criticized historians and "observers" for what he sees as unbridled celebration at the "discovery" of human rights and narratives that suggest "human rights" emerged out of a post-Holocaust global consensus. See Moyn 2010b, 6.

7 Leslie 2019, 192.

8 Anderson 2003, 37.

9 United Nations. 1945. "Charter of the United Nations: Chapter 1 Purposes and Principles." 1945. https://www.un.org/en/sections/un-charter/chapter-i/index .html.

10 United Nations, "The Universal Declaration of Human Rights," 1948. Accessed August 1, 2015. http://www.un.org.

11 United Nations, "Universal Declaration."

12 This language is close to how President Franklin Roosevelt described the four basic freedoms in his 1941 inauguration speech. The speech focused on how the United States could ostensibly protect these freedoms worldwide by entering World War II. See Franklin Delano Roosevelt Presidential Library & Museum 2018.

13 Anderson 2003.

14 NAACP 2009.

15 Anderson 2003, 276.

16 Anderson 2003; Jackson 2007; Somers and Roberts 2008.

17 Leslie 2019.

18 Anderson 2003, 276. Whereas Anderson interprets the NAACP's early campaign for human rights as a genuine attempt by African American leaders to engage with human rights, Moyn (2010b) argues that the brief flirtation with human rights rhetoric by African American leaders such as scholar W. E. B. DuBois was a "second-best strategy" at most (106). Specifically, he argues that leaders' engagement with human rights ended once the anticolonialist campaigns, for which they had invoked human rights in the first place, were thwarted. Thus, Moyn considers achievement of human rights a "last utopia." However, as scholars of Black history and contemporary activists point out, imagining other futures that majority groups perceive as utopian motivates many people of color to social activism. See Kelley 2002 and Walidah Imarisha and adrienne maree brown, *Octavia's Brood: Science Fiction Stories from Social Justice Movements* (Chico, CA: AK Press, 2015).

19 Blain and Gill 2019; Roman 2016.

20 Clapham 2007; Office of the High Commissioner for Human Rights 1996.

21 Romany 1993, 124, fn. 43.

22 Roberts 2014.

23 Jack Donnelly, "The Relative Universality of Human Rights." *Human Rights Quarterly* 29.2 (2007): 281; Pollis 1996.

24 Ignatieff 2009, 4.

25 Vance 1977, 223, emphasis added.

26 Vance 1977, 223.

27 Carter 1979.

28 Mertus 2008.

29 Mertus 2008, 2.

30 Blau et al. 2008.

31 Margaret R. Somers, *Genealogies of Citizenship: Markets, Statelessness, and the Right to Have Rights* (Cambridge: Cambridge University Press, 2008).

32 Berkovitch and Gordon 2016.

33 Stone 2002.

34 As a reminder, the pledge states, "I pledge allegiance to the Flag of the United States of America, and to the Republic for which it stands, one Nation under God, indivisible, with liberty and justice for all." Public school students are required to stand for the Pledge even if they do not recite it.

35 This statement is based on analysis I conducted in 2007. I used a list of state civil rights agencies ("State Civil Rights Offices," FindLaw, http://public.findlaw .com, accessed November 1, 2019). Twenty-one states and Washington, DC, had the phrase "human rights" in their agency title. I then selected one agency from each of the four US census regions and analyzed its website for areas of focus, protected statuses, and mission statement.

36 US Department of State, "Bureau of Democracy, Human Rights, and Labor," accessed August 28, 2017. https://www.state.gov/j/drl/. This is also the page that directly links to www.humanrights.gov.

37 US Department of State, "Under Secretary for Civilian Security, Democracy, and Human Rights," accessed August 28, 2017. https://www.state.gov/j/index .htm.

38 Armaline, Glasberg, and Purkayastha 2011; Blau and Moncada 2006; Hertel and Libal 2011; Merry 2006; Merry et al. 2010; Mertus 2008; Soohoo, Albisa, and Davis 2008; Brunsma, Smith, and Gran 2016.

39 Zoelle 2000.

40 Gallup referred to in Hafner-Burton and Tsutsui 2007.

41 Opportunity Agenda 2007, 2.

42 Opportunity Agenda 2007, 2, emphasis added.

43 Opportunity Agenda 2007, "Project Overview," emphasis added.

44 Opportunity Agenda 2007, 5.

45 Jenkins and Hsu 2008.

46 Hua 2011, 124.

47 Bunch 1995.

48 Meyer et al. 1997, 148.

49 Risse-Kappen, Ropp, and Sikkink 1999.

50 Klug 2005; Sassen 1998.

51 Hafner-Burton and Tsutsui 2005; Tsutsui and Shin 2008; Tustsui, Whitlinger, and Lim 2012.

52 Risse-Kappen, Ropp, and Sikkink 1999.

53 Boutros-Ghali 1999.

54 From the Department of State. Office of Electronic Information, Bureau of Public Affairs 2001a. Also see Department of State. Office of Electronic Information, Bureau of Public Affairs 2001b and the text of First Lady Laura Bush's radio address on the same topic: Bush n.d. Other examples include US-China relations: see CNN 2008.

CHAPTER 2. PUSHED TO HUMAN RIGHTS

1 Thompson 2002.

2 Friedan 1963, 20.

3 Luker 1984.

4 Joffe, Weitz, and Stacey 2004.

5 Hartmann 1987; Silliman and King 1999; and Ziegler 2013.

6   For different takes on Sanger's allying with eugenicists, see Chesler 2007 and Roberts 1997.

7   Roberts 1997.

8   Southern Poverty Law Center 1973.

9   Jessica Luna, "Cross-Cultural Considerations," in *Abortion in the Seventies: Proceedings of the Western Regional Conference on Abortion, Denver, Colorado, February 27–29, 1976*, edited by Warren M. Hern and Bonnie Andrikopoulos, 151–52 (Washington, DC: National Abortion Federation, 1977).

10 While it is beyond the scope of this book, it is important to note that not all illegal abortions were unsafe. Kaplan (1995) documents the history of Jane, a feminist collective that vetted its network of providers. Solinger (2001) has written about how activists for and against abortion rights mobilize the specter of the "back alley butcher" in their political organizing.

11 Luna 1977, 152.

12 In 1977, Hyde proposed a joint resolution (H.J.Res.115): "Joint resolution proposing an amendment to the Constitution of the United States guaranteeing the right of life to the unborn."

13 One state remains in violation of the federal law, whereas others comply with federal law but have additional regulations, such as Iowa, where the governor must approve any Medicaid abortion. About fifteen states fund Medicaid abortion in other cases, some voluntarily, some due to court order. See Guttmacher Institute 2019.

14 Gutiérrez 2008; Schoen 2005.

15 Davis 1981.

16 For more on CARASA and CESA, the Committee to End Sterilization abuse, see Nelson 2003.

17 Rebecca Staton and Meredith Tax of New York City CARASA, Letter to Eleanor Smeal of NOW, August 10, 1978, Loretta Ross papers, Sophia Smith Collection, Smith College, Northampton, Massachusetts.

18 *Harris v. McRae* 1980, emphasis added.

19 *Harris v. McRae* 1980.

20 *Harris v. McRae* 1980, emphasis added.

21 With the fortieth anniversary of the Hyde Amendment falling in a presidential election year, 2016, attention to the budget rider was renewed. Presidential candidate Hillary Clinton called for repeal of the Hyde Amendment, which was a shift for the Democratic Party, which had avoided discussion of reinstituting federal funding for abortion and never previously endorsed overturning it. See Christina Cauterucci, "Why Hillary Clinton's Callout of the Hyde Amendment Is So Important," *Slate*, January 11, 2016.

22 Insurance providers vary on abortion coverage. Also, see Freedman and Stulberg on how increasing Catholic hospital mergers restrict abortion access since various services such as sterilization, miscarriage management, and abortions are not performed at those sites (Freedman and Stulberg 2013). More recent research

shows that patients remain largely unaware of the implications of religious hospital restriction on healthcare and, irrespective of religious background, think it is important patients be informed (Freedman et al. 2018).

23 People of Washington County United for Choice/Wisconsin National Organization for Women, 1981–1983, Reproductive Rights National Network papers, Sophia Smith Collection, Smith College, Northampton, Massachusetts.

24 Buffalo CARASA—Coalition for Abortion Rights and Against Sterilization Abuse, 1980, Reproductive Rights National Network papers, Sophia Smith Collection, Smith College, Northampton, Massachusetts.

25 June K. Inuzuka, "Women of Color and Reproductive Rights," *Pan Asia News*, July/August 1988, SisterSong server.

26 Loretta Ross. Interview by Zakiya Luna, transcript of video recording, May 22, 2006. Global Feminism Project, University of Michigan, https://deepblue.lib.umich.edu/handle/2027.42/55719.

27 National Organization for Women, Women of Color and Reproductive Rights conference flier, 1987, Loretta Ross papers, Sophia Smith Collection, Smith College, Northampton, Massachusetts.

28 Eleanor Smeal of the National Organization for Women in a letter dated January 30, 1987, Loretta Ross papers, Sophia Smith Collection, Smith College, Northampton, Massachusetts.

29 Loretta Ross of the National Organization for Women to Sheri O'Dell and Ellie Smeal, February 11, 1987, Loretta Ross papers, Sophia Smith Collection, Smith College, Northampton, Massachusetts.

30 When we consider that internships in organizations can expand networks and lead to more access to opportunities within a social movement, lower-income women, who are disproportionately women of color, may be systematically excluded from these initial types of opportunities due to their inability to forego payment for labor.

31 Calculated on October 21, 2010, using Bureau of Labor Statistics calculator, the equivalent amount is $48.07. http://data.bls.gov.

32 National Organization for Women, Conference Vignettes, May 27 1987, Loretta Ross papers, Sophia Smith Collection, Smith College, Northampton, Massachusetts. SisterSong newspapers and conferences include the perspectives of women who explicitly identify as pro-life. One column in the *Collective Voices* newspaper was written by a Management Circle member who discussed her opposition to abortion, as stated in the title: "An Anti-Abortionist Surviving in the Pro-Choice Movement" (Skenandore 2004). While SisterSong is formally in support of reproductive options including abortion, it still aims to create a space where ambivalence around these issues can be discussed. SisterSong eventually created a men's caucus and a White allies caucus.

33 Sharon Parker of the National Institute for Women of Color to Loretta Ross, July 25, 1988, Loretta Ross papers, Sophia Smith Collection, Smith College, Northampton, Massachusetts, 01063, emphasis in original.

34 Concerns about cooptation arose in my interviews with RJ activists. See Zakiya T. Luna, "'The Phrase of the Day': Examining Contexts and Co-Optation of Reproductive Justice Activism in the Women's Movement," in *Research in Social Movements, Conflicts, and Change*, vol. 32, edited by Anna Christine Snyder and Stephanie Phetsamay Stobbie, 219–46 (UK: Emerald, 2011).

35 Fried 1990, 6, emphasis in original.

36 Tribe 1990, 177.

37 Bazelon 2010.

38 Daynes and Tatalovich 1992.

39 Saletan 2004.

40 While at the ACLU, Paltrow worked on the case *In re AC*, in which the Court ordered a Caesarian on a woman dying from cancer. See *In re AC* 1987, 533 A. 2d. DC: Court of Appeals. She remained active in reproductive politics, gaining respect as a White ally. She eventually founded National Advocates for Pregnant Women, a legal organization focusing on pregnant women's rights. Paltrow represented people along the political spectrum who had different views on abortion rights, but agreed that people should not lose their autonomy upon becoming pregnant.

41 Luz Alvarez Martinez, interview by Loretta Ross, transcript of video recording, December 6–7, 2004, Voices of Feminism Oral History Project, Sophia Smith Collection, Smith College, Northampton, Massachusetts, 69.

42 Luz Alvarez Martinez, interview by Loretta Ross, transcript of video recording, December 6–7, 2004, Voices of Feminism Oral History Project, Sophia Smith Collection, Smith College, Northampton, Massachusetts, 69–70.

43 Loretta Ross to Jael Silliman et al. 2002, SisterSong papers, Sophia Smith Collection, Smith College, Northampton, Massachusetts.

44 See Mann 2013.

45 For more on Black women and health advocacy, see Smith 2010.

46 Black Women's Health Project, "Legislative Update—April 5th March for Reproductive Freedom Update," *Vital Signs*, Winter 1990—Special Supplement, 3, Black Women's Health Imperative Records, Sophia Smith Collection, Smith College, Northampton, Massachusetts, emphasis added.

47 Flavin 2009; Roberts 1991.

48 Marlene Fried to Loretta Ross, February 27, 1991, Loretta Ross papers, Sophia Smith Collection, Smith College, Northampton, Massachusetts.

49 Murphy traces various organizations that transitioned to research entities that continue to fund population-related projects. See Murphy 2012.

50 Loyd 2014, 176.

51 Loretta Ross to Southeast Women's Health Network, 1991, Loretta Ross papers, Sophia Smith Collection, Smith College, Northampton, Massachusetts; emphasis added.

52 Changed to the Black Women's Health Imperative in 2002.

53 United States Women of Color Delegation to the United Nations Fourth World Conference on Women (USWOCD), U.S. Women of Color Statement

on the Status of Women, August 1995: 5, emphasis added; SisterSong files, Atlanta, GA.

54 Solinger 2001, 5.

55 Luna and Luker 2013.

CHAPTER 3. PULLED TO HUMAN RIGHTS

1 Falcón 2016.

2 Nkenge Touré, interview by Loretta Ross, transcript of video recording, December 4–5, 2004, and March 23, 2005, Voices of Feminism Oral History Project, Sophia Smith Collection, Smith College, Northampton, Massachusetts. Touré eventually secured her General Equivalency Diploma.

3 Nkenge Touré, interview by Loretta Ross.

4 Charon Asetoyer, interview by Joyce Follet, transcript of video recording, September 1–2, 2005, Voices of Feminism Oral History Project, Sophia Smith Collection, Smith College, Northampton, Massachusetts.

5 Luz Alvarez Martinez, interview by Loretta Ross, transcript of video recording, December 6–7, 2004, Voices of Feminism Oral History Project, Sophia Smith Collection, Smith College, Northampton, Massachusetts.

6 Interview by author with NKenge Touré, July 21, 2007, Washington, DC.

7 Interview by author with NKenge Touré.

8 Charlesworth 1995; Sheila Dauer, "Indivisible or Invisible: Women's Human Rights in the Public and Private Sphere," in *Women, Gender, and Human Rights: A Global Perspective*, edited by Marjorie Agosin, 65–82 (New Brunswick, NJ: Rutgers University Press, 2001); Peters and Wolper 1995.

9 Romany 1993, 124.

10 Bunch 1990, 489.

11 MacKinnon 2006.

12 Bunch 1990, 488.

13 Charlesworth 1994, 61.

14 Peters and Wolper 1995, 4.

15 Foerster 2009.

16 Bunch 1990, 491.

17 White, Merrick, and Yazbeck 2006.

18 Every Woman Every Child 2016.

19 A search on the UN website for "contraception" produces multiple pages of results, the first three of which are statistics about contraception use and "unmet need" for contraception. In 2011, the United Nations Population Fund released a report produced in collaboration with the US Center for Reproductive Rights; see United Nations Population Fund 2011. Even though the general UN website "contraception" research results include results from the population, the report is not easy to find, residing instead on the websites of CRR and UNPF.

20 Cook 1995, 256.

21 Turner 2006.

22 Turner 2006, 70.

23 Cook 1995, 256.

24 Ramirez and McEnaney 1997.

25 Merry et al. 2010.

26 Mertus 2008.

27 Merry 2006; Soohoo, Albisa, and Davi 2009.

28 Charon Asetoyer, interview by Joyce Follet, transcript of video recording, September 1–2, 2005, Voices of Feminism Oral History Project, Sophia Smith Collection, Smith College, Northampton, Massachusetts, 85.

29 Dianne Forte Trumpet, *Vital Signs*, Winter 1990, 5, Black Women's Health Imperative Records, Sophia Smith Collection, Smith College, Northampton, Massachusetts.

30 The women were Toni M. Bond, executive director of the Chicago Abortion Fund; Reverend Alma Crawford, Women of Color Partnership of the Religious Coalition for Reproductive Choice; Evelyn S. Field, National Council of Negro Women; Terri James, attorney, American Civil Liberties Union of Illinois; Bisola Marignay, member, National Black Women's Health Project; Cassandra McConnell, Planned Parenthood of Greater Cleveland; Cynthia Newbille, executive director, National Black Women's Health Project; Loretta Ross, Center for Democratic Renewal; Elizabeth Terry, National Abortion Rights Action League of Pennsylvania; "Able" Mable Thomas, Pro-Choice Resource Center, Inc.; Winnette P. Willis, board member, Chicago Abortion Fund; Kim Youngblood, National Black Women's Health Project. Names and affiliations from Toni M. Bond Leonard, "Laying the Foundation for the Reproductive Justice Framework," *Collective Voices* 4.10 (2009). Note that some earlier sources (e.g., Ross 2006) identify this naming as happening *after* Cairo. Retrospectives identify the naming before Cairo. See Ross et al. 2017.

31 Ross 2006, 1.

32 Loretta Ross. Interview by Zakiya Luna, transcript of video recording, May 22, 2006. Global Feminism Project, University of Michigan, https://deepblue.lib.umich.edu/handle/2027.42/55719.

33 As I describe in chapter 5, some activists also used the longer phrase "reproductive social justice." Neither phrase appears in many internal or public documents from SisterSong's early years.

34 Dianne Forte Trumpet, "On the Road to Cairo: African American Women, Population, and Development: A Human Rights Issue." *Vital Signs*, July/August/September 1993, 21, Black Women's Health Imperative Records, Sophia Smith Collection, Smith College, Northampton, Massachusetts.

35 Trumpet, "On the Road to Cairo," 21.

36 United Nations Population Fund 1994, 5.

37 Petchesky 1995; Silliman and King 1999.

38 The Ford Foundation provided funding for some women to attend. Of the twenty-three official women of color delegates to Cairo, five were also involved

in the meetings developing SisterSong. For the National Black Women's Health Project list of "The U.S. Women of Color Delegation Participants," see SisterSong papers, Sophia Smith Collection, Smith College, Northampton, Massachusetts. For decades, the Ford Foundation has funded many organizations, programs, and initiatives. Various activists and scholars question the extent of and the motivations for this funding. Writing on Ford and other philanthropic funders has been relatively limited, perhaps because there is continued reliance on this funding across a range of movement sectors. See Incite! Women of Color Against Violence 2007.

39 Luz Alvarez Martinez, interview by Loretta Ross, transcript of video recording, December 6–7, 2004, Voices of Feminism Oral History Project, Sophia Smith Collection, Smith College, Northampton, Massachusetts, 71–73.

40 A Black Women's Caucus was formed in SNCC in 1968. In 1970, after the caucus had become an independent organization and Puerto Rican women had joined it, the group became the Third World Women's Alliance. See documents formerly available at Women of Color Resource Center's Third World Women's Alliance Archive (http://coloredgirls.live.radicaldesigns.org—last accessed in 2012 but now defunct) and now housed in the Sophia Smith collection at Smith College, Northampton, Massachusetts: https://asteria.fivecolleges.edu. Also see Mohanty 1991, "Introduction" and "Under Western Eyes."

41 Charon Asetoyer, interview by Joyce Follet, transcript of video recording, September 1–2, 2005, Voices of Feminism Oral History Project, Sophia Smith Collection, Smith College, Northampton, Massachusetts, 86–87. In the interview, Asetoyer clarifies that for her "mainstream" denotes "White."

42 Charon Asetoyer, interview by Joyce Follet, 86.

43 National Seminar 1993, 3, emphasis added. Quoted in Rodrigues and Prado 2013, 167.

44 Paxton, Hughes, and Green 2006.

45 Briggs et al. 2013, 111.

46 Sasser 2018.

47 SisterSong, SisterSong Retreat Minutes—Penn Center, South Carolina—November 22–24, 2002, SisterSong papers, Sophia Smith Collection, Smith College, Northampton, Massachusetts.

48 Black Women's Health Project, *Vital Signs*, July/August/September 1994, 18, Black Women's Health Imperative Records, Sophia Smith Collection, Smith College, Northampton, Massachusetts.

49 Women of African Descent for Reproductive Justice to President Clinton, February 21, 1995, SisterSong papers, Sophia Smith Collection, Smith College, Northampton, Massachusetts.

50 Women of African Descent for Reproductive Justice to President Clinton.

51 Specifically, Lani Guinier for Civil Rights Commission and Jocelyn Elders for surgeon general, whose resignation at Clinton's request had left the position open.

52 Bond would later become the SisterSong Management Circle president, a position in which she continued through 2011.

53 There was opposition to holding the conference in China, which many countries and individuals accused of human rights violations. At the time of the conference, the Chinese government held fast to its one-child policy for families in urban areas.

54 Ellen Dorsey, "Center for Democratic Renewal, Letter from the Stanley Foundation to Loretta Ross on Participation in 'Bringing Beijing Back' Conference, Letter," May 31, 1995, Sophia Smith Collection, Smith College, Northampton, Massachusetts.

55 Dorsey, "Center for Democratic Renewal."

56 Dutt 1996, 520.

57 Martinez further reflected on the significance: "And one thing that's also significant is that for the Beijing conference, that was the first time that the document would include women from developed countries, women of color, but nobody knew that we had ever been excluded. They just took it for granted that we were always included and will always be included. So women didn't know that. So I know how important it is to tell that story, what happened in 1994." Luz Alvarez Martinez, interview by Loretta Ross, transcript of video recording, December 6–7, 2004, Voices of Feminism Oral History Project, Sophia Smith Collection, Smith College, Northampton, Massachusetts, 73.

58 USWOCD, *The US Women of Color Statement on the Status of Women*, August 1995, 2, emphasis added.

59 Personal communication with Linda Burnham, University of Michigan Center for Education of Women, 2008 visiting social activist.

60 Mary Chung Hayashi, interview by Loretta Ross, transcript of video recording, December 15, 2006, Voices of Feminism Oral History Project, Sophia Smith Collection, Smith College, Northampton, Massachusetts, 21. In 1993, Hayashi founded the National Asian Women's Health Organization. Hayashi was elected to the California State Assembly in 2006.

61 Silliman et al. 2004, 42.

62 Thomas 2000.

63 Dutt 1996, 520.

CHAPTER 4. TRAINING THE TRAINERS AMIDST BACKLASH

1 SisterSong, "Conf Program_DRAFT," SisterSong server, SisterSong, 14.

2 Hancock 2004; Quadagno 1994; Somers and Block 2005.

3 Levin 2013.

4 Even after TANF was enacted, policies and punishment highly correlated with race of recipient. See Fording, Soss, and Schram 2011.

5 SisterSong Management Circle April 2003 meeting minutes referred to Reform as "deform." SisterSong server. Other organizations used this terminology, too.

6 Collins 2000.

7 Tom Hayden and Dick Flacks, "The Port Huron Statement at 40." *Nation*, July 18, 2002. https://www.thenation.com.

8 Roth 2004.

9 Sara Margaret Evans, *Personal Politics: The Roots of Women's Liberation in the Civil Rights Movement and the New Left* (New York: Vintage, 1979), 238.

10 Robnett 1997.

11 While it may seem obvious that Black women had a central role in the US civil rights movement, Robnett's research was one of the first—if not the first—published social movement studies that questioned the corpus of work by men about the US civil rights movement. See the exchange about Robnett's work in *American Journal of Sociology*, starting with her original article in 1996 followed by a 1997 critique by another scholar and Robnett's reply.

12 Springer 1999, 4.

13 Springer 2005, 3.

14 Roth 2004.

15 Blackwell 2011; Roth 2004.

16 Ferree 2003, 332.

17 Ross in Springer 1999, 4.

18 Beale quoted in Springer 2005, 1.

19 Springer 2005, 63.

20 SisterSong Women of Color Reproductive Health Collective Mission Statement—February 1999, emphasis added, SisterSong server.

21 Ross et al. 2001, 79.

22 Ross et al. 2001, 85.

23 Ross et al. 2001, 85.

24 Ross et al. 2001, 85.

25 SisterSong, "SisterSong: Women of Color Reproductive Health Project Concept Paper Submission April 19, 2001," Sophia Smith Collection, Smith College, Northampton, Massachusetts, 3, emphasis added.

26 SisterSong, "SisterSong: Women of Color Reproductive Health Project," 5.

27 SisterSong, "SisterSong: Women of Color Reproductive Health Project," 5.

28 SisterSong, "SisterSong: Women of Color Reproductive Health Project."

29 SisterSong, "SisterSong Women of Color Reproductive Health Collective Meeting Minutes Alma de Mujer January 25–27, 2002," SisterSong server.

30 SisterSong, "SisterSong Women of Color Reproductive Health Collective Meeting Minutes," SisterSong server, punctuation in original.

31 PDHRE, *The Human Rights Educator* newspaper (December 1996), http://www.pdhre.org.

32 By the end of 1995, the newspaper's circulation was at 2,072,973. *USA Today* n.d.

33 Ross 1996.

34 Ross 1996.

35 SisterSong. "SisterSong: Herstory." *Collective Voices*, 1.2 (2005), 10.
36 Dázon Dixon Diallo interview, transcript of video recording, April 4, 2009, Voices of Feminism Oral History Project, Sophia Smith Collection, Smith College, Northampton, Massachusetts, page 34.
37 Latina Roundtable, Reproductive Health in Women of Color Symposium Agenda, March 1–3, 1997, SisterSong server.
38 Latina Roundtable, notes (in a fax to Jenny Rivera), October 12–14, 1997, Sister-Song server.
39 E-mail from Reena Marcelo, January 13, 1998. SisterSong files, Atlanta, Georgia; all wording, punctuation, and emphasis in the original except for the word "group," for which Marcelo uses "aggrupation."
40 NCHRE, Concept Paper for Participation in the SisterSong: Women of Color Reproductive Health Initiative, SisterSong papers, Sophia Smith Collection, Smith College, Northampton, Massachusetts.
41 NCHRE Odyssey Project Description, Memo, March 16, 1998, SisterSong server.
42 NCHRE Odyssey Project Description, emphasis added.
43 Ford Foundation, letter to Center for Human Rights Education (May 5, 1998), SisterSong papers, Sophia Smith Collection, Smith College, Northampton, Massachusetts.
44 "SisterSong Initial Proposal to Ford for RTIs 1997–2001," SisterSong server.
45 "Latin American" is the phrasing on the original document. "SisterSong Initial Proposal to Ford for RTIs doc 1997–2001," SisterSong server.
46 NCHRE, 1998, "Odyssey Project Description, Memo 3-16-1998" SisterSong papers, Sophia Smith Collection, Smith College, Northampton, Massachusetts.
47 Loretta Ross supported NCHRE by using credit cards linked to her personal account, NCHRE-SS communications folder, SisterSong server.
48 Latina Roundtable (by Luz Rodriguez) to Reena Marcelo of FF, concept paper draft (dated March 30, 1998), SisterSong files, Atlanta, Georgia.
49 SisterSong 6-month progress report Center for Human Rights Education (CHRE) June 1, 1998–December 31, 1998, SisterSong server.
50 NCHRE, Letter from Ross to Luz Rodriguez, October 15, 1998, SisterSong papers, Sophia Smith Collection, Smith College, Northampton, Massachusetts.
51 SisterSong Women of Color Reproductive Health Collective First Collective Training agenda, SisterSong files, Atlanta, Georgia, emphasis added.
52 Luz Rodriguez evaluation, October 27, 1998, SisterSong papers, Sophia Smith Collection, Smith College, Northampton, Massachusetts, emphasis in original.
53 Luz Rodriguez evaluation, October 27, 1998, SisterSong papers, Sophia Smith Collection, Smith College, Northampton, Massachusetts, emphasis in original.
54 Taft 2010.
55 Interview by author with Latonya Slack, May 6, 2009, California.
56 Interview by author with "Jayne," April 1, 2010, California.
57 Hart 2010.

58 During our interview in a semipublic place of Rodriguez's choosing, people stopped by to talk with her. At a different point in the conference when I was talking with Rodriguez, a young organization leader told Rodriguez that sometimes when her small executive committee met, if they had a problem, they would ask themselves, "What would Mama Luz do?" Rodriguez hugged her and told her that she could call at any time.

59 Interview by author with Luz Rodriguez, November 9, 2009, Washington, DC.

60 SisterSong, Canción Latina SisterSong Annual meeting agenda, Atlanta, Georgia May 31, 2000.

61 Puerto Rico is a US territory and thus not technically international. However, territorial residents do not have voting rights like mainland citizens do. Further, at times, SisterSong material referred to the territory using the term "international."

62 Luna 2016.

63 SisterSong, "SisterSong: Women of Color Reproductive Health Project Joint Meeting of Anchor & Anchor Support Committees Savannah, Georgia, September 19–21, 2000, Meeting Minutes, Thursday—September 21, 2000," 5. SisterSong server.

64 Briggs 2003.

65 Tone 2002.

66 NCHRE SisterSong Collective Second Annual Progress Report (Feb. 1, 2000–Jan. 31, 2001), SisterSong files, Atlanta, Georgia.

67 NCHRE SisterSong Collective Third Annual Progress Report (Feb. 1, 2001–June 30, 2001), SisterSong files, Atlanta, Georgia.

68 SisterSong, "Meeting Minutes Alma deMujer January 25–27, 2002," SisterSong server.

69 Roskos 2004.

70 Institute for Women and Ethnic Studies 2001, "Reproductive Health Bill of Rights for Women of Color," SisterSong papers, Sophia Smith Collection, Smith College, Northampton, Massachusetts.

71 Institute for Women and Ethnic Studies 2001, "Reproductive Health Bill of Rights," 1,

72 Institute for Women and Ethnic Studies 2001, "Reproductive Health Bill of Rights," 2.

73 Institute for Women and Ethnic Studies 2001, "Reproductive Health Bill of Rights," 3.

74 Institute for Women and Ethnic Studies 2001, "Reproductive Health Bill of Rights," 16.

75 Cho et al. 2003.

76 Cho et al. 2003.

77 Cho et al. 2003, 4.

78 Cho et al. 2003, 34.

79 Agamben 2008.

80 Ford Foundation 2004.

81 Ford Foundation, "Human Rights and Reproductive Health Committee Update, Memo (10-21-2002)," 1, Sophia Smith Collection, Smith College, Northampton, Massachusetts.

82 Ford Foundation, "Human Rights and Reproductive Health Committee Update," 6.

83 Ford Foundation, "Human Rights and Reproductive Health Committee Update," 2.

84 Ford Foundation, "Human Rights and Reproductive Health Committee Update," 10.

85 Ford Foundation, "Human Rights and Reproductive Health Committee Update," 11, emphasis added.

86 Thomas 2002, i.

87 Thomas 2002, i.

88 Thomas 2002, ii.

89 Thomas, 2002, 10.

90 Thomas 2002, 10.

91 Thomas 2002, 15–16.

92 Philbin 2005.

93 Loretta Ross recommended the book in the Global Feminisms Project interview I conducted in 2006. Cox later wrote an optimistic article about US human rights activism in a law journal—Cox 2008.

94 White, Merrick, and Yazbeck 2006, 10.

95 Bradshaw 2008.

CHAPTER 5. MARCHING TOWARD HUMAN RIGHTS OR REPRODUCTIVE JUSTICE?

1 Staggenborg and Taylor 2005, 45–46.

2 National Organization for Women, "Celebrating Our Presidents," accessed July 23, 2007.

3 National Organization for Women, "March for Women's Lives 1992," emphasis added.

4 National Organization for Women, "History of Marches and Mass Actions," accessed July 23, 2007.

5 National Organization for Women, "History of Marches and Mass Actions," accessed July 23, 2007, emphasis added.

6 Ross/Smeal NOW memo 1987, Sophia Smith Collection, Smith College, Northampton, Massachusetts.

7 Jodi Enda, "Four Major Pro-Choice Groups to March in April," June 13, 2003, http://www.womenenews.org.

8 Amanda Cherrin, "Save Women's Lives: March for Freedom of Choice in 2004." National NOW Times, 2003. http://www.now.org.

9 Amanda Cherrin, "Save Women's Lives."

10 Jodi Enda, "Four Major Pro-Choice Groups to March in April," June 13, 2003, http://www.womenenews.org.

11 Meyer and Corrigall-Brown 2005, 331.

12 Redmond quoted in N'Dieye Gray Danavall and Wavawoman Films, Listen Up! New Voices for Reproductive Justice (Jonesboro, GA: Wavawoman Films, 2005).

13 SisterSong, "Conf program_DRAFT," SisterSong server, 14.

14 SisterSong, "Collective Meeting Spelman College 04–2003 conference brochure event Nov 13–16 2003," SisterSong server.

15 SisterSong, "Conf program_DRAFT," SisterSong server, 28.

16 SisterSong, "Conf program_DRAFT," 28.

17 SisterSong, "Conf program_DRAFT"; see Roberts 1999 on CRACK and its new iteration. See Derkas 2012. The organization still operates today.

18 SisterSong, "Management Circle Meet 2004—Luz Rodriguez' Notes on Minutes of Feb Mtg.doc," emphasis in original, SisterSong server.

19 Nelson 2011; Nelson 2015.

20 Loretta Ross. Interview by Zakiya Luna, transcript of video recording, May 22, 2006. Global Feminism Project, University of Michigan, https://deepblue.lib .umich.edu/handle/2027.42/55719.

21 Barley quoted in N'Dieye Gray Danavall and Wavawoman Films, *Listen Up! New Voices for Reproductive Justice* (Jonesboro, GA: Wavawoman Films, 2005).

22 NCHRE, "New Voices delegation" brochure, SisterSong papers, Sophia Smith Collection, Smith College, Northampton, Massachusetts.

23 At the time, the NOW website included pages archived as far back as 1995, including its newspaper, the *National NOW Times*. This was the first instance of the phrase I found.

24 National Organization for Women, "131 Days until the March for Women's Lives." March News List archives, December 16, 2003 (accessed July 23, 2007).

25 National Organization for Women, "131 Days until the March for Women's Lives." March News List archives, December 16, 2003 (accessed July 23, 2007).

26 Phone interview with author, July 20, 2007, Pennsylvania.

27 Silliman et al. 2004.

28 Loretta Ross, Global Feminisms Project Interview with Loretta Ross, 2006. Video. https://deepblue.lib.umich.edu.

29 Phone interview with author, July 18, 2007, California.

30 SisterSong, Ward/Ross e-mail exchange, 2004, SisterSong papers, Sophia Smith Collection, Smith College, Northampton, Massachusetts.

31 National Organization for Women, March News, March 4, 2004.

32 Smeal quoted in Otis 2004.

33 SisterSong continues to use these signs at events, and pictures of the signs were on the website until a website revision in 2018.

34 SisterSong, "Where Do We Go from Here?" *Collective Voices* 1.1: 2, emphasis added.

35 Loretta Ross. Interview by Zakiya Luna, transcript of video recording, May 22, 2006. Global Feminism Project, University of Michigan, https://deepblue.lib .umich.edu/handle/2027.42/55719.

36 The NOW website was updated since this part of the chapter was written, so the webpages described in this chapter no longer exist. At the time of the initial re-

search, NOW listed twenty-one key issues, including Abortion Rights/Reproductive Issues, Fighting the Right, and Young Feminism. Currently, NOW identifies Reproductive Rights and Justice as one of its six core areas along with Economic Justice (previously Economic Equity), Ending Violence Against Women (previously Violence Against Women), Racial Justice (previously Racial and Ethnic Diversity), LGBTQ Rights (previously Lesbian Rights), and Constitutional Equality (previously listed).

37 Zenaida Mendez, 2006 "Reproductive Justice Is Every Woman's Right." *National NOW Times*, http://www.now.org.

38 Phone interview with author, July 18, 2007, California, emphasis in original.

39 Meyer 2006.

40 SisterSong, "Annual Meeting notes," SisterSong server.

41 Phone interview with author, November 13, 2009, Georgia.

42 Phone interview with author, November 13, 2009, Georgia, emphasis added.

43 SisterSong, "Summary Report Reproductive Justice in the United States: A Funders' Briefing," October 17, 2005, 1, in author's possession.

44 SisterSong, "Summary Report," 2.

45 SisterSong, "Summary Report," 3.

46 SisterSong, "Summary Report," 4.

47 SisterSong, "Summary Report," 4.

48 SisterSong, "Summary Report," 6.

49 SisterSong, "Summary Report," 10.

CHAPTER 6. WRITING RIGHTS AND RESPONSIBILITY

1 When I asked Atlanta office staff about the designation in 2011, they said *membership* status was for women of color–led and –focused organizations (e.g., California Latinas for Reproductive Justice, Tewa Women United) whereas *affiliate* status was for organizations that served women of color but did not have women of color as a focus or in leadership (e.g., National Advocates for Pregnant Women, Planned Parenthood). However, staff also noted that they did not enforce how people designated. For example, the individual membership form allowed people to self-designate. When I answered phones at the office during one data-collection trip, a woman called from Canada asking how to fill out the individual membership form. She explained that she understood the history of women of color and Whites in the United States but since she was Canadian, she was not clear how she was supposed to designate herself. I explained that she could self-select.

2 SisterSong, "Reproductive Rights Are Human Rights." *Collective Voices* 1.3 (2005): 17, emphasis added.

3 Interview with author, March 1, 2020, Georgia.

4 SisterSong, "Reproductive Rights Are Human Rights," 16.

5 SisterSong, "Reproductive Rights Are Human Rights," 16.

6 SisterSong, "Reproductive Rights Are Human Rights," 16.

7   SisterSong, "Reproductive Rights Are Human Rights," 16, emphasis added.

8   Mertus 2008.

9   SisterSong, "Reproductive Rights Are Human Rights," 16, emphasis added.

10 Laura Jiménez, "Ningún Ser Humano Es Ilegal: Immigration Reform, Human Rights, and Reproductive Justice." *Collective Voices* 2.5 (2006): 1–2, emphasis in original.

11 Laura Jiménez, "Ningún Ser Humano Es Ilegal," 1–2, emphasis added.

12 Robin Levi, "Making the Silent Heard and the Invisible Visible: Reproductive Justice for Women in Prison." *Collective Voices* 2.5 (2006): 10.

13 Robin Levi, "Making the Silent Heard," 10.

14 Robin Levi, "Making the Silent Heard," 10.

15 Robin Levi, "Making the Silent Heard," 10.

16 The National Latina Reproductive Health Policy and Justice Advocates, "Latina Mini-Community Update." *Collective Voices* 1.1 (2004): 8, emphasis added.

17 National Latina Reproductive Health Policy and Justice Advocates, "Latina Mini-Community Update," 3, emphasis added.

18 SisterSong, "Building a Movement for Reproductive Justice: An Interview with Loretta Ross." *Collective Voices* 1.2 (2005): 1, emphasis added.

19 Eveline Shen, "Reproductive Justice: Towards a Comprehensive Movement." *Collective Voices* 1.4 (2006): 3, emphasis added.

20 Laura Jiménez, "Ningún Ser Humano Es Ilegal," 1, emphasis added.

21 Brenda Joyner, "Strategizing for the Next Phase of Reproductive Justice." *Collective Voices* 2.7 (2007): 5, emphasis added.

22 Yaminah Ahmad, "Sistersong Creates History." *Collective Voices* 2.7 (2007): 20, emphasis added. The claim beyond "identity and pleasure" is a recognition of critiques of the movement up to that point and is, to some degree, imprecise. The advocacy agenda itself was not explicitly focusing on identity. Still, RJ movement advocates had discussed identity and explained the movement as having been necessary due to experiences resulting from identity-based oppression. Further, the naming of the annual conference—"Let's Talk About Sex!"—and the fact that at each conference opening the Salt 'n' Pepa song of the same name would be played and participants would dance in the aisles were nods to discussion and creation of spaces of pleasure.

23 SisterSong, "Summary Report Reproductive Justice in the United States: A Funders' Briefing." October 17, 2005: 3, emphasis added, in author's possesion.

24 Loretta Ross, "How to Talk about Reproductive Justice." *Collective Voices* 4.10 (2009): 17, emphasis added.

25 Loretta Ross, "How to Talk about Reproductive Justice," 17, emphasis added.

26 Laura Jimènez, "Amnesty for Whom? Abortion as a Human Right; Amnesty International's Big Decision." *Collective Voices* 2.6 (2007): 3.

27 Laura Jimènez, "Amnesty for Whom?" 3, emphasis added.

28 Yaminah Ahmad, "Prisons Shackle Women Inmates in Labor." *Collective Voices* 2.6 (2007): 12.

29 NCHRE, "New Voices delegation" brochure, SisterSong papers, Sophia Smith Collection, Smith College, Northampton, Massachusetts.

30 SisterSong, "SisterSong Post-Conference Report." *Collective Voices* 1.1 (2004): 11–12.

31 SisterSong, "SisterSong Post-Conference Report," 11.

32 SisterSong, "SisterSong Post-Conference Report," 12, emphasis added.

33 SisterSong, "SisterSong Post-Conference Report," 12, emphasis added.

34 Leila Hessini, "Globalizing Radical Agendas: How US Policies Affect Women's Reproductive Rights around the World." *Collective Voices* 1.1 (2004).

35 Leila Hessini, "Globalizing Radical Agendas."

36 Ayesha M. Imam, "Women's Reproductive and Sexual Rights in the Offence of Zina in Muslim Laws in Nigeria." *Collective Voices* 2.5 (2006).

37 Leila Hessini, "Strategies of Resistance: Women Re-Interpreting the Meaning of Democracy in the Arab World." *Collective Voices* 2.6 (2007).

38 Lynn Roberts, "Mobilizing Support for Community Health Workers in Trinidad." *Collective Voices* 2.6 (2007).

39 Leila Hessini, "Strategies of Resistance."

40 SisterSong, "Beijing + 10: U.S. Proposed Amendment Defeated." *Collective Voices* 1.3 (2005).

41 Ross 2006, 6.

42 SisterSong, "ReproMujeresDeColore2004FinalDraft," SisterSong server.

43 Choo and Ferree 2010.

44 Falcón 2016.

45 Falcón 2016, 129.

46 Loretta Ross. Interview by Zakiya Luna, transcript of video recording, May 22, 2006. Global Feminism Project, University of Michigan, https://deepblue.lib .umich.edu/handle/2027.42/55719.

47 SisterSong, "Reproductive Justice 101: Atlanta," e-mail, September 12, 2007, in author's possession.

48 Images of the quilt appeared in later conference programs and in advertising. The Global Feminism Project used an image of the quilt in an issue of *Feminist Studies* (36.1, Spring 2010) that featured a set of articles on the project.

49 Universal Declaration of Human Rights booklet.

50 PowerPoint slides from a 2007 RJ 101 presentation, October 20, 2007, Atlanta, GA.

51 Taylor 1996.

52 Roberts 2014, 178.

53 PowerPoint slides from a 2007 RJ 101 presentation, October 20, 2007, Atlanta, GA. These specific slides were also part of other presentations like one titled "Self-Help and Reproductive Justice rev LJ 5-22-2006." "LJ" indicates that Laura Jimenez revised the presentation.

54 Luft and Ward 2009; Choo and Ferree 2010.

55 PowerPoint slides from a 2009 RJ 102 presentation, SisterSong organizational files, Atlanta GA.

56 Rosenberg 1991.

57 Choo and Ferree 2010; Cole 2009; Crenshaw 1991; McCall 2005.

CHAPTER 7. "THEY'RE ALL INTERTWINED"

1 In other chapters, I include examples of skeptics who, for varying reasons, questioned the utility of human rights.

2 Interview with author, November 9, 2009, New York.

3 Lewis, Aydin, and Powell 2017.

4 The United Nations foundation estimated in 2016 that its student events reached twenty-six thousand people between middle school and college. http://www .unausa.org/membership. There is a hope that the launch of a free mobile application, MyDiplomat, will expose more young people to the UN and offer a different way to engage in Model UN. https://unausa.org/model-un/.

5 Interview with author, August 7, 2009, California.

6 Mertus 2008.

7 Phone interview with author, July 18, 2007, California.

8 Dudziak 2003.

9 Phone interview with author, December 7, 2009, US South.

10 Interview with author, October 26 2009, Georgia.

11 Phone interview with author, July 20, 2007, Virginia.

12 Interview with author, February 22, 2010, Georgia.

13 Interview with author, March 1 and 3, 2010, Georgia.

14 Interview with author, August 7, 2009, California, emphasis added.

15 Interview with author, November 9, 2009, New Mexico.

16 Phone interview with author, July 31, 2009, emphasis added.

17 Interview with author, February 25, 2010, Georgia.

18 Phone interview with author, July 20, 2007, Virginia.

19 Phone interview with author, November 30, 2009, California.

20 Phone interview with author, October 8, 2009, Texas.

21 Phone interview with author, July 27, 2009, Washington, DC, emphasis added.

22 Phone interview with author, August 17, 2007, Washington, DC, emphasis added.

23 Phone interview with author, July 5, 2007.

24 Phone interview with author, September 11, 2010, Illinois.

25 Interview with author, August 7, 2009, California, emphasis added.

26 Interview with author, February 23, 2010, Georgia.

27 Interview with author, November 9, 2009, New York, emphasis added.

28 Interview with author, October 26 2009, Georgia, emphasis added

29 Phone interview with author, April 3, 2010, Iowa.

30 Phone interview with author, July 31, 2009, Illinois.

31 Interview with author, March 16, 2010, Michigan.

32 Interview with author, February 25, 2010, Georgia.

33 Phone interview with author, July 20, 2007, Pennsylvania.

34 Phone interview with author, December 10, 2009, Pennsylvania.

35 Phone interview with author, December 10, 2009, Pennsylvania.

36 She specifically referenced the poster being from Syracuse Cultural Workers. "Laminated Poster—Universal Declaration of Human Rights," Syracuse Cultural Workers, accessed November 2, 2019. https://www.syracuseculturalworkers.

37 Mertus 2008, 230.

38 Waltz 2001, 44.

39 Ewick and Silbey 1998, 20.

40 Ewick and Silbey 1998, 20.

41 Ewick and Silbey 1998.

CHAPTER 8. "PUPPIES AND RAINBOWS" OR PRAGMATIC POLITICS?

1 Roberts 2014.

2 In her 2016 book *Power Interrupted*, Sylvanna Falcón examines the process leading up to and at the 2011 World Conference on Racism. She cites several examples of how the US delegation appeared to engage in a "campaign to disrupt and obstruct" (110).

3 US Department of State, Report of the United States of America Submitted to the UN High Commissioner for Human Rights in Conjunction with the Universal Periodic Review, 2010.

4 Center for Reproductive Rights et al. 2010, 1.

5 "Human Rights Kowtow" 2010.

6 US Department of State 2011b, emphasis added.

7 Rudiger 2011.

8 Mertus 2008, 160.

9 Abrams 2012.

10 For example, see Williams 2013.

11 Fetner 2008.

12 Human Rights Campaign, http://www.hrc.org, Initial access 2008, last accessed 2016.

13 Farmer 2005, 9.

14 Phone interview with author, July 5, 2007, Washington, DC.

15 Phone interview with author, June 18, 2007, New York.

16 Phone interview with author, September 1, 2009, Colorado.

17 Phone interview with author, April 16, 2010, Oregon; referring to the Strong Families campaign, https://forwardtogether.org.

18 Phone interview with author, July 20, 2007, Virginia, emphasis added.

19 Interview with author, November 9, 2009, Washington, DC.

20 Interview with author, November 9, 2009, Washington, DC.

21 For arguments about employer cost savings, see Cynthia Dailard, "The Cost of Contraceptive Insurance Coverage." *Guttmacher Policy Review* 6.1 (2003): 12–13.

A National Public Radio story highlights the effectiveness of this type of argument by detailing an exchange in which a Republican legislator is impressed by data showing cost savings. See Rovner 2012. For one example of the persistence of these arguments, see the Power to Decide website. It is a rebranding of the National Campaign to Prevent Unplanned Pregnancy, which focuses on teen pregnancy. A webpage specifically connects reduced births and taxes: "Thanks to young people, the United States has made historic progress in helping match young people's intentions and actions regarding pregnancy—the teen birth rate plummeted by 64% between 1991 and 2015. This progress thus far creates *$4.4 billion in public savings each year*, according to new analyses by Power to Decide" (Power to Decide: The Campaign to Prevent Unplanned Pregnancy n.d., emphasis added). Also see Advocates for Youth n.d.

22 Kingdon 2011.

23 Kingdon 2011, 1.

24 Both progressive and conservative thinkers use "poverty pimp" to denote people whose paid work relies on studying poverty or working with people in poverty. Generally, a "poverty pimp" is more interested in personal gain than in changing conditions of poverty. Stanford economics professor and noted conservative Tomas Sowell published "The Poverty Pimp's Poem"—Sowell 2001. For academic discussion see Diversi and Finley 2010.

25 Luna 2016.

26 For the text of the amendment, see "Amendment to H.R.," United States House of Representatives, 2009, http://housedocs.house.gov.

27 Christian Davenport, Sarah A. Soule, and David A. Armstrong, "Protesting While Black? The Differential Policing of American Activism, 1960 to 1990." *American Sociological Review* 76.1 (2011): 152–78.

28 American Civil Liberties Union 2009.

29 SisterSong, "Top-line talking points," in author's possession.

30 Interview with author, February 24, 2010, Georgia.

31 SisterSong, "Top-line talking points," in author's possession.

32 After the Stupak Amendment passed, Stupack responded to critics who raised concerns regarding the class implications of the amendment. He stated, "If current law is a class divide, then they [opponents] must conclude that current law is too. No, all I'm doing is keeping current law—I'm not trying to divide classes or anything like that. All I'm doing is keeping current law that's been current law since 1976." The current law referred to was the Hyde Amendment, which eliminated federal funding for abortion barring exceptional circumstances such as provable rape. Good 2009.

33 Interview with author, February 25, 2010, Georgia.

34 Interview with author, February 23, 2010, Georgia, emphasis added.

35 Interview with author, February 23, 2010, Georgia. For academic analyses, see Richie et al. 2012 and Luna 2017.

36 For additional analyses, see Richie et al. 2012 and Luna 2017.
37 Quadagno 1994; Suzanne Mettler, *The Submerged State: How Invisible Government Policies Undermine American Democracy* (Chicago: University of Chicago Press, 2011).
38 Blee 2012, 82.
39 SisterSong Women of Color Reproductive Health Collective Mission Statement—February 2005, emphasis added, SisterSong server.
40 SisterSong Women of Color Reproductive Health Collective Mission Statement—November 1999, emphasis added, SisterSong server.
41 SisterSong homepage, www.sistersong.net, July 25, 2016.

CONCLUSION

 1 SisterSong homepage, www.sistersong.net, February 16, 2016, emphasis added.
 2 Stammers 1999, 1006.
 3 Brown 1992, 8.
 4 Bogost 2012; Morton 2010.
 5 Todd 2016.
 6 Todd 2016.
 7 Pinn 2017.
 8 Hua 2011, 124.
 9 Nigatu and Clayton n.d.
10 Dutt 1996, 520.
11 Gomez and Wapman 2017.
12 Cole 2012; Hafner-Burton and Tsutsui 2005; Tsutsui, Whitlinger, and Lim 2012.
13 Ford 2019.
14 Ford 2019.
15 Ferree 2003, 340.
16 Interview with author, February 24, 2010, Georgia.
17 Harris-Perry 2016.
18 The Women's March Organizers and Condé Nast 2018.
19 Black Mamas Matter Alliance, "Black Maternal Health Week," Black Mamas Matter Alliance, accessed September 24, 2019, https://blackmamasmatter.org.
20 Pew Research Center, "Public Opinion on Abortion." *Pew Research Center's Religion & Public Life Project* (blog), August 29, 2019, https://www.pewforum.org/fact-sheet/public-opinion-on-abortion.
21 *SisterSong v. Kemp* 2019.
22 Associated Press 2019.
23 Luna 2018.
24 American Civil Liberties Union 2019, emphasis added.
25 *SisterSong v. Kemp* 2019, 6.
26 Ericka Huggins, Lecture on "Identity, Activism, and Change." AS Program Board and Black Student Union, University of California, Santa Barbara, February 21, 2019.

APPENDIX A

1 Lofland 1996, 43.
2 Lofland 1996.
3 Yin 2003.
4 Social movement organizations produce a wealth of artifacts, but analysis of artifacts is more common in anthropology (see Yin 2003).
5 Melissa Murray and Kristin Luker, *Cases on Reproductive Rights and Justice* (Foundation Press, 2015).
6 Patricia Hill Collins, "Learning from the Outsider Within: The Sociological Significance of Black Feminist Thought." *Social Problems* 33.6 (1986): S14–32.
7 Julia Sudbury and Margo Okazawa-Rey, *Activist Scholarship: Antiracism, Feminism, and Social Change* (London: Pluto Press, 2009); Patricia Hill Collins, *On Intellectual Activism* (Philadelphia: Temple University Press, 2012).

REFERENCES

Abrams, Jim. 2012. "Senate Takes Up UN Disability Treaty." Yahoo! News, November 12. https://news.yahoo.com.

Advocates for Youth. N.d. "Teenage Pregnancy, the Case for Prevention: An Updated Analysis of Recent Trends and Federal Expenditures Associated with Teenage Pregnancy." Advocates for Youth. Accessed April 9, 2018. http://www.advocatesforyouth .org.

Agamben, Giorgio. 2008. *State of Exception*. Chicago: University of Chicago Press.

Agosin, Marjorie. 2001. *Women, Gender, and Human Rights: A Global Perspective*. New Brunswick, NJ: Rutgers University Press.

Althusser, Louis. 1970. "Ideology and Ideological State Apparatuses (Notes towards an Investigation)." In *Lenin and Philosophy and Other Essays*, translated by Ben Brewster, 127–86. New York: Monthly Review Press.

American Civil Liberties Union. 2009. "The Stupak-Pitts Amendment." American Civil Liberties Union, December 2. https://www.aclu.org.

———. 2019. "ACLU Files Lawsuit Challenging Georgia Abortion Ban." American Civil Liberties Union, June 28. https://www.aclu.org.

Anderson, Carol. 2003. *Eyes off the Prize: African Americans, the United Nations, and the Struggle for Human Rights, 1944–1955*. New York: Cambridge University Press.

Anzaldúa, Gloria. 1990. *Making Face, Making Soul/Haciendo Caras: Creative and Critical Perspectives by Feminists of Color*. San Francisco: Aunt Lute Books.

Armaline, William T., and Davita Silfen Glasberg. 2009. "What Will States Really Do for Us? The Human Rights Enterprise and Pressure from Below." *Societies without Borders* 4 (3): 430–51. https://doi.org/10.1163/187188609X12492771031771.

Armaline, William T., Davita Silfen Glasberg, and Bandana Purkayastha. 2011. *Human Rights in Our Own Backyard: Injustice and Resistance in the United States*. Vol. 1. Pennsylvania Studies in Human Rights. Philadelphia: University of Pennsylvania Press.

———. 2017. "De Jure vs. de Facto Rights: A Response to 'Human Rights; What the United States Might Learn from the Rest of the World and, Yes, from American Sociology.'" *Sociological Forum* 32 (1): 220–24. https://doi.org/10.1111/socf.12303.

Armstrong, Elizabeth A. 2002. *Forging Gay Identities: Organizing Sexuality in San Francisco, 1950–1994*. Chicago: University of Chicago Press.

Associated Press. 2019. "Restrictive Georgia Abortion Law Target of ACLU, Planned Parenthood Lawsuit." *USA Today*, July 23. https://www.usatoday.com.

Balkin, J. M. 2005. *What Roe V. Wade Should Have Said: The Nation's Top Legal Experts Rewrite America's Most Controversial Decision*. New York: NYU Press.

Baumgardner, Jennifer, and Amy Richards. 2000. *Manifesta: Young Women, Feminism, and the Future*. New York: Macmillan.

Bazelon, Emily. 2010. "The New Abortion Providers." *New York Times*, July 18. http://www.nytimes.com.

Berkovitch, Nitza, and Neve Gordon. 2016. "Differentiated Decoupling and Human Rights." *Social Problems* 63 (4): 499–512. https://doi.org/10.1093/socpro/spw020.

Bernstein, Mary. 2005. "Identity Politics." *Annual Review of Sociology* 31 (1): 47–74.

Bernstein, Mary, and Nancy A. Naples. 2015. "Altared States: Legal Structuring and Relationship Recognition in the United States, Canada, and Australia." *American Sociological Review* 80 (6): 1226–49. https://doi.org/10.1177/0003122415613414.

Blackwell, Maylei. 2011. *¡Chicana Power! Contested Histories of Feminism in the Chicano Movement*. Austin: University of Texas Press.

Blain, Keisha, and Tiffany Gill. 2019. *To Turn the Whole World Over: Black Women and Internationalism*. Champaign: University of Illinois Press.

Blau, Judith. 2016. "Human Rights: What the United States Might Learn from the Rest of the World and, Yes, from American Sociology." *Sociological Forum* 31 (4): 1126–39. https://doi.org/10.1111/socf.12299.

———. 2017. "Human Rights Matter." *Sociological Forum* 32 (1): 225–27. https://doi.org/10.1111/socf.12304.

Blau, Judith R., David L. Brunsma, Alberto Moncada, and Catherine Zimmer. 2008. *The Leading Rogue State: The United States and Human Rights*. Boulder, CO: Paradigm.

Blau, Judith R., and Alberto Moncada. 2006. *Justice in the U.S.: Human Rights and the U.S. Constitution*. Lanham, MD: Rowman & Littlefield.

———. 2007. "Sociologizing Human Rights: Reply to John Hagan and Ron Levi." *Sociological Forum* 22 (3): 381.

Blee, Kathleen M. 2012. *Democracy in the Making: How Activist Groups Form*. New York: Oxford University Press.

Bogost, Ian. 2012. *Alien Phenomenology; or, What It's Like to Be a Thing*. Minneapolis: University of Minnesota Press.

Boutros-Ghali, Boutros. 1999. *Unvanquished, a United Nations–United States Saga*. London: Tauris.

Bradshaw, Sarah. 2008. "Is the Rights Focus the Right Focus? Nicaraguan Responses to the Rights Agenda." In *The Politics of Rights: Dilemmas for Feminist Praxis*, edited by Andrea Cornwall and Maxine Molyneux, 155–67. London: Routledge.

Briggs, Laura. 2003. *Reproducing Empire: Race, Sex, Science, and U.S. Imperialism in Puerto Rico*. Berkeley: University of California Press.

Briggs, Laura, Faye Ginsburg, Elena R. Gutiérrez, Rosalind Petchesky, Rayna Rapp, Andrea Smith, and Chikako Takeshita. 2013. "Roundtable: Reproductive Technologies and Reproductive Justice." *Frontiers: A Journal of Women Studies* 34 (3): 102–25.

Brown, Wendy. 1992. "Finding the Man in the State." *Feminist Studies* 18 (1): 7–34.

Brunsma, David L., Keri E. Iyall Smith, and Brian K. Gran. 2015. *Handbook of Sociology and Human Rights.* New York: Routledge.

———. 2016. *Institutions Unbound: Social Worlds and Human Rights.* New York: Routledge.

Buck v. Bell. 1927, 274 US 200. Supreme Court.

Bunch, Charlotte. 1990. "Women's Rights as Human Rights: Toward a Re-Vision of Human Rights." *Human Rights Quarterly* 12 (4): 486–98.

———. 1995. "Transforming Human Rights from a Feminist Perspective." In *Women's Rights, Human Rights: International Feminist Perspectives,* edited by Julie Stone Peters and Andrea Wolper, 11–17. New York: Routledge.

Bush, Laura. N.d. "Laura Bush: The Weekly Address Delivered by the First Lady." The American Presidency Project, UC–Santa Barbara. Accessed February 28, 2018. http://www.presidency.ucsb.edu/ws/?pid=24992.

Carragee, Kevin M., and Wim Roefs. 2004. "The Neglect of Power in Recent Framing Research." *Journal of Communication* 54 (2): 214–33. https://doi.org/10.1111/j.1460-2466.2004.tb02625.x.

Carter, James. 1979. "Jimmy Carter: Atlanta, Georgia, Remarks Accepting the Martin Luther King, Jr. Nonviolent Peace Prize." The American Presidency Project, USC–Santa Barbara, January 14. http://www.presidency.ucsb.edu.

Center for Reproductive Rights, SisterSong Women of Color Reproductive Justice Collective, Rebecca Project for Human Rights, Law Students for Reproductive Justice, National Asian Pacific American Women's Forum, National Abortion Federation, and Women on the Rise Telling HerStory. 2010. "Report on the United States' Compliance with Its Human Rights Obligations in the Area of Women's Reproductive and Sexual Health." Center for Reproductive Rights. https://www.reproductiverights.org.

Center for Women's Global Leadership. N.d. "Activist Origins of the Campaign." Center for Women's Global Leadership. Accessed October 18, 2018. https://16dayscwgl.rutgers.edu.

Charlesworth, Hilary. 1994. "What Are 'Women's International Human Rights'?" In *Human Rights of Women: National and International Perspectives,* edited by Rebecca J. Cook, 58–84. Philadelphia: University of Pennsylvania Press.

———. 1995. "Women's Human Rights: The Emergence of a Movement." In *Women's Rights, Human Rights: International Feminist Perspectives,* edited by Julie Stone Peters and Andrea Wolper, 103–13. New York: Routledge.

Cheng, Sealing. 2011. "The Paradox of Vernacularization: Women's Human Rights and the Gendering of Nationhood." *Anthropological Quarterly* 84 (2): 475–505.

Chesler, Ellen. 2007. *Woman of Valor: Margaret Sanger and the Birth Control Movement in America.* New York: Simon & Schuster.

Cho, Eunice, Lisa Crooms, Heidi Dorow, Andy Huff, Ethel Long Scott, and Dorothy Q. Thomas. 2003. "Something Inside So Strong: A Resource Guide on Human Rights in the United States." US Human Rights Network. https://www.ushrnetwork.org.

Choo, Hae Yeon, and Myra Marx Ferree. 2010. "Practicing Intersectionality in Sociological Research: A Critical Analysis of Inclusions, Interactions, and Institutions in the Study of Inequalities." *Sociological Theory* 28 (2): 129–49. https://doi .org/10.1111/j.1467-9558.2010.01370.x.

Clapham, Andrew. 2007. *Human Rights: A Very Short Introduction*. Very Short Introductions. New York: Oxford University Press.

Clay, Andreana. 2012. *The Hip-Hop Generation Fights Back: Youth, Activism, and Post–Civil Rights Politics*. New York: NYU Press.

Clément, Dominique. 2015. "The Sociology of Human Rights." *Canadian Journal of Sociology* 40 (4): 563–65.

CNN. 2008. "Bush Chides China over Human Rights—CNN.Com." *Politics* (blog). August 7, 2008. http://edition.cnn.com/2008/POLITICS/08/06/bush.china.olympics /index.html.

Cole, Elizabeth R. 2009. "Intersectionality and Research in Psychology." *American Psychologist* 64 (3): 170–80. http://dx.doi.org/10.1037/a0014564.

Cole, Elizabeth R., and Zakiya T. Luna. 2010. "Making Coalitions Work: Solidarity across Difference within US Feminism." *Feminist Studies* 36 (1): 71.

Cole, Wade M. 2012. "A Civil Religion for World Society: The Direct and Diffuse Effects of Human Rights Treaties, 1981–2007." *Sociological Forum* 27 (4): 937–60. https://doi.org/10.1111/j.1573-7861.2012.01363.x.

Collins, Patricia Hill. 2000. *Black Feminist Thought: Knowledge, Consciousness, and the Politics of Empowerment*. Rev. 10th anniversary edition. New York: Routledge.

Collins, Patricia Hill, and Sirma Bilge. 2016. *Intersectionality*. Hoboken, NJ: Wiley.

Combahee River Collective. 1983. "Combahee River Collective Statement." In *Home Girls: A Black Feminist Anthology*, edited by Barbara Smith, 272–82. New York: Kitchen Table: Women of Color Press.

Cook, Rebecca. 1995. "International Human Rights and Women's Reproductive Health." In *Women's Rights, Human Rights: International Feminist Perspectives*, edited by Julie Stone Peters and Andrea Wolper, 256–75. New York: Routledge.

Cottrell, Debbie Mauldin. 2010. "National Women's Conference, 1977." Texas State Historical Association, June 15. https://tshaonline.org.

Cox, Larry. 2008. "A Movement for Human Rights in the United States: Reasons for Hope." *Columbia Human Rights Law Review* 40 (Fall): 135–47.

Crenshaw, Kimberlé. 1989. "Demarginalizing the Intersection of Race and Sex: A Black Feminist Critique of Antidiscrimination Doctrine, Feminist Theory, and Antiracist Politics." *University of Chicago Legal Forum* 1989: 139.

———. 1991. "Mapping the Margins: Intersectionality, Identity Politics, and Violence against Women of Color." *Stanford Law Review* 43 (6): 1241–99.

Davis, Angela Y. 1981. *Women, Race, and Class*. Vol. 1. New York: Random House.

Daynes, Byron W., and Raymond Tatalovich. 1992. "Presidential Politics and Abortion, 1972–1988." *Presidential Studies Quarterly* 22 (3): 545–61.

Department of State. The Office of Electronic Information, Bureau of Public Affairs. 2001a. "Executive Summary." U.S. Department of State Archives, November 17. https://2001-2009.state.gov.state.gov, in author's possession.

———. 2001b. "Report on the Taliban's War against Women." U.S. Department of State Archives, November 17. https://2001-2009.state.gov, in author's possession.

Derkas, Erica. 2012. "The Organization Formerly Known as CRACK: Project Prevention and the Privatized Assault on Reproductive Wellbeing." *Race, Gender, and Class* 19 (3): 179.

Diversi, Marcelo, and Susan Finley. 2010. "Poverty Pimps in the Academy: A Dialogue about Subjectivity, Reflexivity, and Power in Decolonizing Production of Knowledge." *Cultural Studies ↔ Critical Methodologies* 10 (1): 14–17. https://doi.org/10.1177/1532708609351147.

Donnelly, Jack. 2007. *International Human Rights*. Vol. 3. Dilemmas in World Politics. Boulder, CO: Westview.

Dudziak, Mary L. 2003. "The Supreme Court's History of Indifference to the Opinions of Other Countries' Courts." History News Network, Columbian College of Arts & Sciences, September 22. https://historynewsnetwork.org/article/1693.

Dutt, Mallika. 1996. "Some Reflections on U.S. Women of Color and the United Nations Fourth World Conference on Women and NGO Forum in Beijing, China." *Feminist Studies* 22 (3): 519–28.

Emerson, Robert M., Rachel I. Fretz, and Linda L. Shaw. 1995. *Writing Ethnographic Fieldnotes*. Chicago: University of Chicago Press.

Eschle, Catherine. 2002. "Engendering Global Democracy." *International Feminist Journal of Politics* 4 (3): 315.

Every Woman Every Child. 2016. "The Global Strategy for Women's, Children's, and Adolescents' Health." UNICEF. https://data.unicef.org.

Ewick, Patricia, and Susan S. Silbey. 1998. *The Common Place of Law: Stories from Everyday Life*. Language and Legal Discourse. Chicago: University of Chicago Press.

Falcón, Sylvanna M. 2016. *Power Interrupted: Antiracist and Feminist Activism inside the United Nations*. Seattle: University of Washington Press.

Farmer, Ashley D. 2017. "The Third World Black Woman, 1970–1979." In *Remaking Black Power: How Black Women Transformed an Era*, 159–92. Chapel Hill: University of North Carolina Press. https://www.jstor.org.

Farmer, Paul. 2005. *Pathologies of Power: Health, Human Rights, and the New War on the Poor*. Berkeley: University of California Press.

Feminist Studies. 2010. Special issue on *Rethinking the Global*, 36 (1). Accessed January 14, 2019. http://www.feministstudies.org.

Ferree, Myra Marx. 2003. "Resonance and Radicalism: Feminist Framing in the Abortion Debates of the United States and Germany." *American Journal of Sociology* 109 (2): 304.

Ferree, Myra Marx, William Anthony Gamson, Jürgen Gerhards, and Dieter Rucht. 2002. *Shaping Abortion Discourse: Democracy and the Public Sphere in Germany and the United States*. New York: Cambridge University Press.

Fetner, Tina. 2008. *How the Religious Right Shaped Lesbian and Gay Activism*. Minneapolis: University of Minnesota Press.

Finnegan, Amy C., Adam P. Saltsman, and Shelley K. White. 2010. "Negotiating Politics and Culture: The Utility of Human Rights for Activist Organizing in the United States." *Journal of Human Rights Practice* 2 (3): 307–33. https://doi.org/10.1093/jhuman/huq009.

Flavin, Jeanne. 2009. *Our Bodies, Our Crimes: The Policing of Women's Reproduction in America*. Alternative Criminology Series. New York: NYU Press.

Foerster, Amy. 2009. "Contested Bodies." *International Feminist Journal of Politics* 11 (2): 151–73. https://doi.org/10.1080/14616740902789500.

Ford Foundation. 2002. "A Revolution of the Mind: Funding Human Rights in the United States." New York: Ford Foundation.

———. 2004. "Close to Home: Case Studies of Human Rights Work in the United States." New York: Ford Foundation.

Ford, Liz. 2019. "UN Waters Down Rape Resolution to Appease US's Hardline Abortion Stance." *Guardian*, April 23, sec. global development. https://www.theguardian.com.

Fording, Richard C., Joe Soss, and Sanford F. Schram. 2011. "Race and the Local Politics of Punishment in the New World of Welfare." *American Journal of Sociology* 116 (5): 1610–57. https://doi.org/10.1086/657525.

Foundation Center. N.d. "Humanrights2015_highlights.Pdf." Foundations Center. Accessed July 27, 2015. http://foundationcenter.org.

Franklin Delano Roosevelt Presidential Library & Museum. 2018. "FDR and the Four Freedoms Speech." Franklin Delano Roosevelt Presidential Library & Museum. https://fdrlibrary.org.

Fraser, Arvonne. 1999. "Becoming Human: The Origins and Development of Women's Human Rights." *Human Rights Quarterly* 21 (4): 853–906.

Fraser, Nancy. 1997. *Justice Interruptus: Critical Reflections on the "Postsocialist" Condition*. New York: Psychology Press.

Freedman, Lori R., Luciana E. Hebert, Molly F. Battistelli, and Debra B. Stulberg. 2018. "Religious Hospital Policies on Reproductive Care: What Do Patients Want to Know?" *American Journal of Obstetrics and Gynecology* 218 (2): 251.e1–251.e9. https://doi.org/10.1016/j.ajog.2017.11.595.

Freedman, Lori R., and Debra B. Stulberg. 2013. "Conflicts in Care for Obstetric Complications in Catholic Hospitals." *AJOB Primary Research* 4 (4): 1–10. https://doi.org/10.1080/21507716.2012.751464.

Fried, Marlene Gerber. 1990. *From Abortion to Reproductive Freedom: Transforming a Movement*. Vol. 1. Boston: South End Press.

George, Sheba, Nelida Duran, and Keith Norris. 2013. "A Systematic Review of Barriers and Facilitators to Minority Research Participation among African Americans,

Latinos, Asian Americans, and Pacific Islanders." *American Journal of Public Health* 104 (2): e16–31. https://doi.org/10.2105/AJPH.2013.301706.

Gibson, James L. 2004. "Truth, Reconciliation, and the Creation of a Human Rights Culture in South Africa." *Law & Society Review* 38 (1): 5–40.

Gomez, Anu Manchikanti, and Mikaela Wapman. 2017. "Under (Implicit) Pressure: Young Black and Latina Women's Perceptions of Contraceptive Care." *Contraception* 96 (4): 221–26. https://doi.org/10.1016/j.contraception.2017.07.007.

Good, Chris. 2009. "Stupak on the Stupak Amendment." *Atlantic*, November 12. https://www.theatlantic.com.

Gutiérrez, Elena R. 2008. *Fertile Matters: The Politics of Mexican-Origin Women's Reproduction*. Vol. 1. Chicana Matters Series. Austin: University of Texas Press. http://www.loc.gov.

Guttmacher Institute. 2019. "State Funding of Abortion under Medicaid." Guttmacher Institute, August 1. https://www.guttmacher.org.

Hafner-Burton, Emilie M., and Kiyoteru Tsutsui. 2005. "Human Rights in a Globalizing World: The Paradox of Empty Promises." *American Journal of Sociology* 110 (5): 1373–1411.

———. 2007. "Justice Lost! The Failure of International Human Rights Law to Matter Where Needed Most." *Journal of Peace Research* 44 (4): 407–25. https://doi.org/10.1177/0022343307078942.

Halfmann, Drew. 2011. *Doctors and Demonstrators: How Political Institutions Shape Abortion Law in the United States, Britain, and Canada*. Chicago: University of Chicago Press.

Hancock, Ange-Marie. 2004. *The Politics of Disgust: The Public Identity of the Welfare Queen*. New York: NYU Press.

Harris v. McRae. 1980, 448 US 297. Supreme Court.

Harris-Perry, Melissa. 2016. "24 Books, Essays, and Other Texts to Read Because You're Still Having Trouble Processing the Election." *Elle*, November 29. https://www.elle.com.

Hart, Randle J. 2010. "There Comes a Time: Biography and the Founding of a Movement Organization." *Qualitative Sociology* 33 (1): 55–77. https://doi.org/10.1007/s11133-009-9135-3.

Hartmann, Betsy. 1987. *Reproductive Rights and Wrongs: The Global Politics of Population Control and Contraceptive Choice*. Vol. 1. New York: Harper & Row.

Heinz, Eric. 2007. "Truth and Myth in Critical Race Theory and Latcrit: Human Rights and the Ethnocentrism of Anti-Ethnocentrism." *National Black Law Journal* 20: 107–62.

Hertel, Shareen, and Kathryn Libal. 2011. *Human Rights in the United States: Beyond Exceptionalism*. New York: Cambridge University Press.

Hertel, Shareen, Lyle Scruggs, and C. Patrick Heidkamp. 2009. "Human Rights and Public Opinion: From Attitudes to Action." *Political Science Quarterly* 124 (3): 443–59. https://doi.org/10.1002/j.1538-165X.2009.tb00655.x.

Heywood, Leslie, and Jennifer Drake. 1997. *Third Wave Agenda: Being Feminist, Doing Feminism*. Minneapolis: University of Minnesota Press.

Hsu, Andrea. 2010. "Difficult Births: Laboring and Delivering in Shackles." *All Things Considered*. National Public Radio. https://www.npr.org.

Hua, Julietta. 2011. *Trafficking Women's Human Rights*. Minneapolis: University of Minnesota Press.

"Human Rights Kowtow." 2010. *Wall Street Journal*, August, 24. http://online.wsj.com.

Hunt, Lynn Avery. 2007. *Inventing Human Rights: A History*. New York: Norton.

Hunt, Scott, Robert D. Benford, and David A. Snow. 1994. "Identity Fields: Framing Processes and the Social Construction of Movement Identities." In *New Social Movements: From Ideology to Identity*, edited by Enrique Larana, Hank Johnston, and Joseph R. Gusfield, 185–208. Philadelphia: Temple University Press.

Ignatieff, Michael. 2009. *American Exceptionalism and Human Rights*. Princeton, NJ: Princeton University Press.

In re AC. 1987, 533 A. 2d. DC: Court of Appeals.

Incite! Women of Color Against Violence. 2007. *The Revolution Will Not Be Funded: Beyond the Non-Profit Industrial Complex*. Boston: South End Press.

Inuzuka, June K. 1991. "Women of Color and Public Policy: A Case Study of the Women's Business Ownership Act." *Stanford Law Review* 43 (6): 1215–39. https://doi.org/10.2307/1229038.

Ishay, Micheline. 2008. *The History of Human Rights: From Ancient Times to the Globalization Era*. Berkeley: University of California Press.

Jackson, Thomas F. 2007. *From Civil Rights to Human Rights: Martin Luther King, Jr., and the Struggle for Economic Justice*. Philadelphia: University of Pennsylvania Press.

Jenkins, Alan, and Kevin Shawn Hsu. 2008. "American Ideals & Human Rights: Findings from New Public Opinion Research by the Opportunity Agenda." *Fordham Law Review* 77: 439.

Joffe, Carole, Tracy Weitz, and C. L. Stacey. 2004. "Uneasy Allies: Pro-Choice Physicians, Feminist Health Activists, and the Struggle for Abortion Rights." *Sociology of Health & Illness* 26 (6): 775–96. https://doi.org/10.1111/j.0141-9889.2004.00418.x.

Kaplan, Laura. 1995. *The Story of Jane: The Legendary Underground Feminist Abortion Service*. New York: Pantheon.

Kelley, Robin D. G. 2002. *Freedom Dreams: The Black Radical Imagination*. Boston: Beacon.

Kerr, Joanna. 1993. *Ours by Right: Women's Rights as Human Rights*. London: Zed.

King, Deborah K. 1988. "Multiple Jeopardy, Multiple Consciousness: The Context of a Black Feminist Ideology." *Signs* 14 (1): 42–72.

Kingdon, John W. 2011. *Agendas, Alternatives, and Public Policies*. Harlow, UK: Longman.

Klug, Heinz. 2005. "Transnational Human Rights: Exploring the Persistence and Globalization of Human Rights." *Annual Review of Law and Social Science* 1 (1): 85–103. https://doi.org/10.1146/annurev.lawsocsci.1.041604.115903.

Labaton, Vivien, and Dawn Lundy Martin. 2009. *The Fire This Time: Young Activists and the New Feminism*. New York: Knopf Doubleday.

Lader, Lawrence. 1974. *Abortion II: Making the Revolution*. Boston: Beacon.

Landy, David. 2013. "Talking Human Rights: How Social Movement Activists Are Constructed and Constrained by Human Rights Discourse." *International Sociology* 28 (4): 409–28. https://doi.org/10.1177/0268580913490769.

Leslie, Grace V. 2019. "'United, We Build a Free World': The Internationalism of Mary McLeod Bethune and the National Council of Negro Women." In *To Turn the Whole World Over: Black Women and Internationalism*, edited by Keisha N. Blain and Tiffany M. Gill, 192–218. Black Internationalism. Chicago: University of Illinois Press. https://www.jstor.org.

Levin, Josh. 2013. "The Real Story of Linda Taylor, America's Original Welfare Queen." *Slate*, December 19. http://www.slate.com.

Levitsky, Sandra R. 2007. "Niche Activism: Constructing a Unified Movement Identity in a Heterogeneous Organizational Field." *Mobilization: An International Journal* 12 (3): 271–86.

Levitt, Peggy, and Sally Merry. 2009. "Vernacularization on the Ground: Local Uses of Global Women's Rights in Peru, China, India, and the United States." *Global Networks* 9 (4): 441–61. https://doi.org/10.1111/j.1471-0374.2009 .00263.x.

Lewis, John, Andrew Aydin, and Nate Powell. 2017. "March: Congressman John Lewis, Andrew Aydin, and Nate Powell in Conversation." Presented at the Los Angeles Times Festival of Books, Los Angeles, CA, April 22. https://festivalofbooks2017 .sched.com.

Lofland, John. 1996. *Social Movement Organizations: Guide to Research on Insurgent Realities*. Social Problems and Social Issues. New York: de Gruyter.

Lofland, John, David Snow, Leon Anderson, and Lyn H. Lofland. 2006. *Analyzing Social Settings: A Guide to Qualitative Observation and Analysis*. Belmont, CA: Wadsworth/Thomson.

Loyd, Jenna M. 2014. *Health Rights Are Civil Rights: Peace and Justice Activism in Los Angeles, 1963–1978*. Minneapolis: University of Minnesota Press.

Luft, Rachel E., and Jane Ward. 2009. "Toward an Intersectionality Just out of Reach: Confronting Challenges to Intersectional Practice." *Advances in Gender Research* 13 (June): 9–37. https://doi.org/10.1108/S1529-2126(2009)0000013005.

Luker, Kristin. 1984. *Abortion and the Politics of Motherhood*. California Series on Social Choice and Political Economy. Berkeley: University of California Press.

Luna, Jessica. 1977. "Cross-Cultural Considerations." In *Abortion in the Seventies: Proceedings of the Western Regional Conference on Abortion, Denver, Colorado, February 27–29, 1976*, edited by Warren M. Hern and Bonnie Andrikopoulos, 151–52. Washington, DC: National Abortion Federation.

Luna, Zakiya. 2016. "'Truly a Women of Color Organization': Negotiating Sameness and Difference in Pursuit of Intersectionality." *Gender & Society* 30 (5): 769–90. https://doi.org/10.1177/0891243216649929.

———. 2017. "Who Speaks for Whom? (Mis) Representation and Authenticity in Social Movements." *Mobilization: An International Quarterly* 22 (4): 435–50. https://doi .org/10.17813/1086-671X-22-4-435.

———. 2018. "'Black Children Are an Endangered Species': Examining Racial Framing in Social Movements." *Sociological Focus* 51 (3): 238–51. https://doi.org/10.1080/0038 0237.2018.1412233.

Luna, Zakiya, and Kristin Luker. 2013. "Reproductive Justice." *Annual Review of Law and Social Science* 9 (1): 327–52. https://doi.org/10.1146/annurev-lawsocsci -102612-134037.

MacKinnon, Catharine A. 2006. *Are Women Human? And Other International Dialogues.* Cambridge, MA: Belknap Press of Harvard University Press.

Mann, Emily S. 2013. "Regulating Latina Youth Sexualities through Community Health Centers: Discourses and Practices of Sexual Citizenship." *Gender & Society* 27 (5): 681–703. https://doi.org/10.1177/0891243213493961.

Mansbridge, Jane J., and Aldon D. Morris. 2001. *Oppositional Consciousness: The Subjective Roots of Social Protest.* Chicago: University of Chicago Press.

McCall, Leslie. 2005. "The Complexity of Intersectionality." *Signs: Journal of Women in Culture and Society* 30 (3): 1771–1800.

Melucci, Alberto. 1994. "A Strange Kind of Newness: What's 'New' in New Social Movements?" In *New Social Movements: From Ideology to Identity*, edited by Enrique Larana, Hank Johnston, and Joseph R. Gusfield, 101–30. Philadelphia: Temple University Press. http://muse.jhu.edu/book/9620.

Merry, Sally Engle. 2006. *Human Rights and Gender Violence: Translating International Law into Local Justice.* Chicago: University of Chicago Press.

Merry, Sally Engle, Peggy Levitt, Mihaela Çerban Rosen, and Diana H. Yoon. 2010. "Law from Below: Women's Human Rights and Social Movements in New York City." *Law & Society Review* 44 (1): 101–28.

Mertus, Julie. 2008. *Bait and Switch: Human Rights and U.S. Foreign Policy.* Vol. 2. Global Horizons Series. New York: Routledge.

Meyer, David S. 2006. "Claiming Credit: Stories of Movement Influence as Outcomes." *Mobilization: An International Quarterly* 11 (3): 281–98.

Meyer, David S., and Catharine Corrigall-Brown. 2005. "Coalitions and Political Context: U.S. Movements against Wars in Iraq." *Mobilization: An International Journal* 10 (3): 327–44.

Meyer, John W., John Boli, George M. Thomas, and Francisco O. Ramirez. 1997. "World Society and the Nation-State." *American Journal of Sociology* 103 (1): 144–81. https:// doi.org/10.1086/231174.

Mohanty, Chandra Talpade, Ann Russo, and Lourdes Torres. 1991. *Third World Women and the Politics of Feminism.* Bloomington: Indiana University Press.

Morton, Timothy. 2010. *The Ecological Thought.* Cambridge, MA: Harvard University Press.

Moyn, Samuel. 2010a. "Human Rights in History." *Nation*, August 11. https://www .thenation.com.

———. 2010b. *The Last Utopia: Human Rights in History.* Cambridge, MA: Belknap Press of Harvard University Press.

Murphy, Michelle. 2012. *Seizing the Means of Reproduction: Entanglements of Feminism, Health, and Technoscience.* Durham, NC: Duke University Press.

NAACP (National Association for the Advancement of Colored People). 2009. "World War II and the Post War Years—NAACP: A Century in the Fight for Freedom." Exhibitions—Library of Congress. Webpage, February 21. https://www.loc.gov.

National Committee for Responsive Philanthropy. N.d. "Freedom Funders." *National Committee for Responsive Philanthropy* (blog). Accessed January 17, 2019. https://www.ncrp.org/publication/freedom-funders.

Nelson, Alondra. 2011. *Body and Soul: The Black Panther Party and the Fight against Medical Discrimination.* Minneapolis: University of Minnesota Press.

Nelson, Jennifer. 2003. *Women of Color and the Reproductive Rights Movement.* New York: NYU Press.

———. 2015. *More Than Medicine: A History of the Feminist Women's Health Movement.* New York: NYU Press.

Nigatu, Heben, and Tracy Clayton. 2017, April 26. "Episode 89: Sister Girl Bonds (with Dr. Kimberle Crenshaw)." Another Round. Accessed May 6, 2017. https://www.acast.com.

Office of the High Commissioner for Human Rights. 1996. "Fact Sheet No.2 (Rev.1): The International Bill of Human Rights." Office of the High Commissioner for Human Rights..http://www.ohchr.org.

Okamoto, Dina G. 2003. "Toward a Theory of Panethnicity: Explaining Asian American Collective Action." *American Sociological Review* 68 (6): 811–42. https://doi.org/10.2307/1519747.

Opportunity Agenda. 2007. *Human Rights in the U.S.: Opinion Research with Advocates, Journalists, and the General Public.* Washington, DC: Opportunity Agenda.

Otis, Ginger Adams. 2004. "Racism and Reproductive Rights." *Nation*, April 22. http://www.thenation.com.

Paxton, Pamela, Melanie M. Hughes, and Jennifer L. Green. 2006. "The International Women's Movement and Women's Political Representation, 1893–2003." *American Sociological Review* 71 (6): 898–920. https://doi.org/10.1177/000312240607100602.

Pearce, Tola Olu. 2001. "Human Rights and Sociology: Some Observations from Africa." *Social Problems* 48 (1, 50th Anniversary Issue): 48–56.

Petchesky, Rosalind Pollack. 1995. "From Population Control to Reproductive Rights: Feminist Fault Lines." *Reproductive Health Matters* 3 (6): 152–61. https://doi.org/10.1016/0968-8080(95)90172-8.

Peters, Julie Stone, and Andrea Wolper. 1995. "Introduction." In *Women's Rights, Human Rights: International Feminist Perspectives*, edited by Julie Stone Peters and Andrea Wolper, 1–8. New York: Routledge.

Philbin, Marianne. 2005. "Close to Home: Bringing Human Rights to Illinois." Loretta Ross papers. Sophia Smith Archive, Smith College Libraries, Northampton, Massachusetts.

Pinn, Anthony. 2017. *When Colorblindness Isn't the Answer: Humanism and the Challenge of Race.* Durham, NC: Pitchstone.

Polletta, Francesca, and James M. Jasper. 2001. "Collective Identity and Social Movements." *Annual Review of Sociology* 27: 283.

Pollis, Adamantia. 1996. "Cultural Relativism Revisited: Through a State Prism." *Human Rights Quarterly* 18 (2): 316–44.

Power to Decide: The Campaign to Prevent Unplanned Pregnancy. N.d. "Progress Pays Off." Power to Decide. Accessed April 9, 2018. https://powertodecide.org.

Price, Kimala. 2010. "What Is Reproductive Justice? How Women of Color Activists Are Redefining the Pro-Choice Paradigm." *Meridians: Feminism, Race, Transnationalism* 10 (2): 42–65.

Quadagno, Jill S. 1994. *The Color of Welfare: How Racism Undermined the War on Poverty.* New York: Oxford University Press.

Ramirez, Francisco O., and Elizabeth H. McEnaney. 1997. "From Women's Suffrage to Reproduction Rights? Cross-National Considerations." *International Journal of Comparative Sociology* 38 (1/2): 6.

Reese, Ellen, and Garnett Newcombe. 2003. "Income Rights, Mothers' Rights, or Workers' Rights? Collective Action Frames, Organizational Ideologies, and the American Welfare Rights Movement." *Social Problems* 50 (2): 294–318.

Richie, Beth E., Dana-Ain Davis, and LaTosha Traylor. 2012. "Feminist Politics, Racialized Imagery, and Social Control." *Souls* 14 (1–2): 54–66. https://doi.org/10.1080/109 99949.2012.723407.

Risse-Kappen, Thomas, Steve C. Ropp, and Kathryn Sikkink. 1999. *The Power of Human Rights: International Norms and Domestic Change.* Vol. 66. Cambridge Studies in International Relations. Cambridge: Cambridge University Press.

Roberts, Christopher N. J. 2014. *The Contentious History of the International Bill of Human Rights.* New York: Cambridge University Press.

———. 2017. "Human Rights and Sociological Duties." *Sociological Forum* 32 (1): 213–16. https://doi.org/10.1111/socf.12301.

Roberts, Dorothy E. 1991. "Punishing Drug Addicts Who Have Babies: Women of Color, Equality, and the Right of Privacy." *Harvard Law Review* 104 (7): 1419–82. https://doi.org/10.2307/1341597.

———. 1997. *Killing the Black Body: Race, Reproduction, and the Meaning of Liberty.* New York: Vintage Books.

Robinson, B. A. N.d. "Pledge of Allegiance" Accessed September 11, 2018. http://www .religioustolerance.org.

Robnett, Belinda. 1997. *How Long? How Long? African-American Women in the Struggle for Civil Rights.* New York: Oxford University Press.

Rodrigues, Cristiano, and Marco Aurelio Prado. 2013. "A History of the Black Women's Movement in Brazil: Mobilization, Political Trajectory, and Articulations with the State." *Social Movement Studies* 12 (2): 158–77. http://dx.doi.org/10.1080/16121 97X.2012.697613.

Roe v. Wade. 1973, 410 US 113. Supreme Court.

Roman, Meredith. 2016. "The Black Panther Party and the Struggle for Human Rights." *Spectrum: A Journal on Black Men* 5 (1): 7–32.

Romany, Celina. 1993. "Women as Aliens: A Feminist Critique of the Public/Private Distinction in International Human Rights Law." *Harvard Human Rights Journal* 6: 87–125.

Rosen, Mihaela Şerban, and Diana H. Yoon. 2009. "'Bringing Coals to Newcastle'? Human Rights, Civil Rights, and Social Movements in New York City." *Global Networks* 9 (4): 507–28. https://doi.org/10.1111/j.1471-0374.2009.00266.x.

Rosenberg, Gerald N. 1991. *The Hollow Hope: Can Courts Bring About Social Change?* American Politics and Political Economy Series. Chicago: University of Chicago Press.

Roskos, Laura H. 2004. "From the Center to the Margins: The Radicalization of Human Rights in the United States." *Meridians* 4 (2): 129–36.

Ross, Loretta. 1996. "Stop Talking and Finish Women's Treaty." *USA Today*, September 27. Access World News (Formerly America's Newspapers).

———. 2006. "Understanding Reproductive Justice." SisterSong Women of Color Reproductive Health Collective. http://www.sistersong.net.

Ross, Loretta, J. Brownlee, Sarah L. Brownlee, Dázon Dixon Diallo, Luz Rodriguez, and Latina Roundtable. 2001. "The SisterSong Collective: Women of Color, Reproductive Health, and Human Rights." *American Journal of Health Studies* 17 (2): 79–88.

Ross, Loretta, Erika Derkas, Whitney Peoples, Lynn Roberts, and Pamela Bridgewater. 2017. *Radical Reproductive Justice: Foundation, Theory, Practice, Critique*. New York: Feminist Press at CUNY.

Roth, Benita. 2004. *Separate Roads to Feminism: Black, Chicana, and White Feminist Movements in America's Second Wave*. New York: Cambridge University Press.

Rovner, Julie. 2012. "How Birth Control Saves Taxpayers Money." National Public Radio, March 6. https://www.npr.org.

Rudiger, Anja. 2011. "Hypocrisy on Human Rights: Obama Administration Offers Words but No Action on Economic and Social Rights." *Huffington Post* (blog), March 21. http://www.huffingtonpost.com/anja-rudiger/hypocrisy-on-human-rights_b_837728.html.

Rudy, Kathy. 2000. "Difference and Indifference: A U.S. Feminist Response to Global Politics." *Signs* 25 (4): 1051–53.

Russo, Ann. 2006. "The Feminist Majority Foundation's Campaign to Stop Gender Apartheid." *International Feminist Journal of Politics* 8 (4): 557–80. https://doi.org/10.1080/14616740600945149.

Saletan, William. 2004. *Bearing Right: How Conservatives Won the Abortion War*. Berkeley: University of California Press.

Sassen, Saskia. 1998. *Globalization and Its Discontents: Essays on the New Mobility of People and Money*. New York: New Press.

Sasser, Jade S. 2018. *On Infertile Ground: Population Control and Women's Rights in the Era of Climate Change*. New York: NYU Press.

Schoen, Johanna. 2005. *Choice and Coercion: Birth Control, Sterilization, and Abortion in Public Health and Welfare.* Chapel Hill: University of North Carolina Press.

Silliman, Jael M., Marlene Gerber Fried, Loretta Ross, and Elena R. Gutierrez. 2004. *Undivided Rights: Women of Color Organize for Reproductive Justice.* Boston: South End Press.

Silliman, Jael Miriam, and Ynestra King. 1999. *Dangerous Intersections: Feminist Perspectives on Population, Environment, and Development.* Boston: South End Press.

SisterSong v. Kemp. 2019. United States District Court for the Northern District of Georgia Atlanta Division, Docket 1:19-cv-02973-SCJ, https://www.aclu.org/cases/sistersong-v-kemp.

SisterSong Women of Color Reproductive Health Collective. 2003. "SisterSong—Women of Color Reproductive Health Collective." Internet Archive, June 19. https://web.archive.org.

———. 2014. "SisterSong Is Building a Movement for Reproductive Justice." Internet Archive, June 3. https://web.archive.org.

Sjoberg, Gideon, Elizabeth A. Gill, and Norma Williams. 2001. "A Sociology of Human Rights." *Social Problems* 48 (1): 11–47. https://doi.org/10.1525/sp.2001.48.1.11.

Skenandore, Alice. 2004. "An Anti-Abortionist Surviving in the Pro-Choice Movement." *Collective Voices* 1 (1): 3.

Smeal, Eleanor, and Helen Cho. 2009. "Why Is the Feminist Majority Foundation Refusing to Abandon the Women and Girls of Afghanistan?" *Huffington Post* (blog), July 15. http://www.huffingtonpost.com/eleanor-smeal/why-is-the-fmf-refusing-t_b_234595.html.

Smith, Andrea. 2007. "Social Justice Activism in the Academic Industrial Complex." *Journal of Feminist Studies in Religion* 23 (2): 140–45.

Smith, Susan. 2010. *Sick and Tired of Being Sick and Tired: Black Women's Health Activism in America, 1890–1950.* Philadelphia: University of Pennsylvania Press.

Snow, David A., and Robert D. Benford. 1992. "Master Frames and Cycles of Protest." In *Frontiers in Social Movement Theory*, edited by Aldon D. Morris and Carol McClurg Mueller, 133–55. New Haven, CT: Yale University Press.

Snow, David A., E. Burke Rochford, Steven K. Worden, and Robert D. Benford. 1986. "Frame Alignment Processes, Micromobilization, and Movement Participation." *American Sociological Review* 51 (4): 464–81. https://doi.org/10.2307/2095581.

Solinger, Rickie. 2001. *Beggars and Choosers: How the Politics of Choice Shapes Adoption, Abortion, and Welfare in the United States.* Vol. 1. New York: Hill and Wang.

Somers, Margaret R. 2008. *Genealogies of Citizenship: Markets, Statelessness, and the Right to Have Rights.* Cambridge University Press.

Somers, Margaret R., and Fred Block. 2005. "From Poverty to Perversity: Ideas, Markets, and Institutions over 200 Years of Welfare Debate." *American Sociological Review* 70 (2): 260–87.

Somers, Margaret R., and Christopher N. J. Roberts. 2008. "Toward a New Sociology of Rights: A Genealogy of 'Buried Bodies' of Citizenship and Human Rights." *Annual Review of Law and Social Science* 4: 385–425.

Soohoo, Cynthia. 2008. "Introduction: Close to Home; Social Justice Activism and Human Rights." *Columbia Human Rights Law Review* 40 (1): 7–17.

Soohoo, Cynthia, Catherine Albisa, and Martha F. Davis. 2009. *Bringing Human Rights Home: A History of Human Rights in the United States*. Philadelphia: University of Pennsylvania Press.

Southern Poverty Law Center. 1973. Relf v. Weinberger. Southern Poverty Law Center. http://www.splcenter.org.

Sowell, Thomas. 2001. "The Poverty Pimp's Poem." *Capitalism*, June 11. https://www.capitalismmagazine.com.

Springer, Kimberly. 1999. *Still Lifting, Still Climbing: African American Women's Contemporary Activism*. New York: NYU Press.

———. 2005. *Living for the Revolution: Black Feminist Organizations, 1968–1980*. Durham, NC: Duke University Press.

Staggenborg, Suzanne, and Verta Taylor. 2005. "Whatever Happened to the Women's Movement?" *Mobilization: An International Quarterly* 10 (1): 37–52. https://doi.org/10.17813/maiq.10.1.46245r7082613312.

Stammers, Neil. 1999. "Social Movements and the Social Construction of Human Rights." *Human Rights Quarterly* 21 (4): 980–1008. https://doi.org/10.1353/hrq.1999.0054.

Steinberg, M. W. 1999. "The Talk and Back Talk of Collective Action: A Dialogic Analysis of Repertoires of Discourse among Nineteenth-Century English Cotton Spinners." *American Journal of Sociology* 105 (3): 736. https://doi.org/10.1086/210359.

Steinman, Erich. 2012. "Settler Colonial Power and the American Indian Sovereignty Movement: Forms of Domination, Strategies of Transformation." *American Journal of Sociology* 117 (4): 1073–1130. https://doi.org/10.1086/662708.

Stern, Alexandra Minna. 2005. *Eugenic Nation: Faults and Frontiers of Better Breeding in Modern America*. Berkeley: University of California Press.

Stone, Adam. 2002. "Human Rights Education and Public Policy in the United States: Mapping the Road Ahead." *Human Rights Quarterly* 24 (2): 537–57. https://doi.org/10.1353/hrq.2002.0029.

Taft, Jessica K. 2010. *Rebel Girls: Youth Activism and Social Change across the Americas*. New York: NYU Press.

Targeted News Service. 2013. "Human Rights Council Holds Annual Full-Day Discussion on Women's Human Rights." UC–Santa Barbara Library, June 5. http://infoweb.newsbank.com.proxy.library.ucsb.edu.

Taylor, Verta A. 1996. *Rock-a-by Baby: Feminism, Self-Help, and Postpartum Depression*. Perspectives on Gender. New York: Routledge.

Taylor, Verta, and Nancy E. Whittier. 1992. "Collective Identity in Social Movement Communities: Lesbian Feminist Mobilization." In *Frontiers in Social Movement Theory*, edited by Aldon D. Morris and Carol McClurg Mueller, 104–29. New Haven, CT: Yale University Press.

The Women's March Organizers, and Condé Nast. 2018. *Together We Rise: Behind the Scenes at the Protest Heard around the World*. New York: HarperCollins. https://www.harpercollins.com.

Thomas, Dorothy Q. 2000. "We Are Not the World: U.S. Activism and Human Rights in the Twenty-First Century." *Signs: Journal of Women in Culture and Society* 25 (4): 1121. https://doi.org/doi:10.1086/495530.

———. 2002. "Revolution of the Mind: Funding Human Rights in the United States (a Report to the Ford Foundation)." Loretta Ross papers. Sophia Smith Archive, Smith College, Northampton, Massachusetts.

Thompson, Becky. 2002. "Multiracial Feminism: Recasting the Chronology of Second Wave Feminism." *Feminist Studies* 28 (2): 336–60.

Todd, Zoe. 2016. "An Indigenous Feminist's Take on the Ontological Turn: 'Ontology' Is Just Another Word for Colonialism." *Journal of Historical Sociology* 29 (1): 4–22. https://doi.org/10.1111/johs.12124.

Tone, Andrea. 2002. *Devices and Desires: A History of Contraceptives in America*. New York: Macmillan.

Tribe, Laurence H. 1990. *Abortion: The Clash of Absolutes*. Vol. 1. New York: Norton.

Tsutsui, Kiyoteru, and Hwa Ji Shin. 2008. "Global Norms, Local Activism, and Social Movement Outcomes: Global Human Rights and Resident Koreans in Japan." *Social Problems* 55 (3): 391–418. https://doi.org/10.1525/sp.2008.55.3.391.

Tsutsui, Kiyoteru, Claire Whitlinger, and Alwyn Lim. 2012. "International Human Rights Law and Social Movements: States' Resistance and Civil Society's Insistence." *Annual Review of Law and Social Science* 8 (1): 367–96. https://doi.org/10.1146/annurev-lawsocsci-102811-173849.

Turner, Bryan S. 2006. *Vulnerability and Human Rights*. Essays on Human Rights. University Park: Pennsylvania State University Press.

United Nations. 1945. "Charter of the United Nations: Chapter 1, Purposes and Principles." United Nations, June 17. https://www.un.org.

United Nations. Division for the Advancement of Women. 2000. *Bringing International Human Rights Law Home: Judicial Colloquium on the Domestic Application of the Convention on the Elimination of All Forms of Discrimination against Women and the Convention on the Rights of the Child*. New York: United Nations.

United Nations Population Fund. 1994. "Programme of Action of the Conference (94/5/12)." United Nations Population Fund, May 12. http://www.un.org.

———. 2011. "The Rights to Contraceptive Information and Services for Women and Adolescents." United Nations Population Fund. https://www.un.org.

———. 2014. "Cairo, Programme of Action, 20th Anniv, English.pdf." United Nations Population Fund. http://www.unfpa.org.

United States. Congress. Senate. Committee on Foreign Relations. 1991. "Convention on the Elimination of All Forms of Discrimination against Women." *S. Hrg.* 101–1119: 109.

United States. Congress. Senate. Committee on Foreign Relations. Subcommittee on International Operations. 2000. *The United Nations: Progress in Promoting U.S. Interests: Hearing before the Subcommittee on International Operations of the Committee on Foreign Relations, United States Senate, One Hundred Sixth*

Congress, First Session, November 3, 1999. Washington, DC: Government Printing Office.

United States. Congress. Senate. Council on Foreign Relations. Committee on Foreign Relations and United Nations Security Council. 2000. *The Future of U.S.-U.N. Relations: A Dialogue between the U.S. Senate Committee on Foreign Relations and the U.N. Security Council.* Washington, DC: Government Printing Office.

US Department of State. 1996. "May 1996 Report: Follow-up to 4WCW." May. US Department of State. https://1997-2001.state.gov.

———. 2010. "Report of the United States of America Submitted to the U.N. High Commissioner for Human Rights in Conjunction with the Universal Periodic Review." US Department of State. https://www.state.gov.

———. 2011a. "Report of the Working Group on the Universal Periodic Review United States of America." US Department of State. https://www.state.gov.

———. 2011b. "U.S. Response to UN Human Rights Council Working Group Report." US Department of State, March 10. http://www.state.gov.

———. N.d. "Bureau of Democracy, Human Rights, and Labor." US Department of State. Accessed August 28, 2017. https://www.state.gov.

———. N.d. "Under Secretary for Civilian Security, Democracy, and Human Rights." US Department of State. Accessed August 28, 2017. https://www.state.gov.

———. N.d. "Universal Periodic Review." US Department of State. Accessed April 20, 2018. https://www.state.gov/j/drl/upr/index.htm.

———. N.d. "Universal Periodic Review Process." US Department of State. Accessed April 20, 2018. https://www.state.gov.

US Human Rights Network. 2003. "Something Inside So Strong: A Resource Guide on Human Rights in the United States." US Human Rights Network, December 10. http://www.ushrnetwork.org.

USA Today. N.d. "About *USA Today* Timeline." USA Today. Accessed July 24, 2019. https://www.usatoday.com.

Van Dyke, Nella, Sarah A. Soule, and Verta A. Taylor. 2004. "The Targets of Social Movements: Beyond a Focus on the State." In *Authority in Contention*, 25: 27–51. Research in Social Movements, Conflicts, and Change 25. Bingley, UK: Emerald Group. http://www.emeraldinsight.com.

Vance, Cyrus. 1977. "Human Rights and Foreign Policy." Presented at the Law Day Address, Lumpkin School of Law, University of Georgia, April 30. Reprinted in Cyrus Vance, "Human Rights and Foreign Policy." *Georgia Journal of International and Comparative Law* 7 (1997): 223–29.

Wade, Lisa. 2011. "Loretta Ross on the Phrase 'Women of Color.'" Sociological Images. *Loretta Ross on the Phrase "Women of Color"* (blog), March 26. https://thesoci etypages.org/socimages/2011/03/26/loreta-ross-on-the-phrase-women-of-color/.

Walker, Rebecca. 1995. *To Be Real: Telling the Truth and Changing the Face of Feminism.* New York: Anchor Books.

Waltz, Susan. 2001. "Universalizing Human Rights: The Role of Small States in the Construction of the Universal Declaration of Human Rights." *Human Rights Quarterly* 23 (1): 44–72.

Washington, Harriet A. 2006. *Medical Apartheid: The Dark History of Medical Experimentation on Black Americans from Colonial Times to the Present*. New York: Doubleday.

Western States Center. 2011. *The Origin of the Phrase "Women of Color."* https://www.youtube.com/watch?v=82vl34mi4Iw.

White, Arlette Campbell, Thomas William Merrick, and Abdo Yazbeck. 2006. *Reproductive Health: The Missing Millennium Development Goal: Poverty, Health, and Development in a Changing World*. Washington, DC: World Bank.

Williams, Vanessa. 2013. "To Critics, Obama's Scolding Tone with Black Audiences Is Getting Old." *Washington Post*, May 20, sec. Style. https://www.washingtonpost.com.

Yin, Robert K. 2003. *Case Study Research: Design and Methods*. Thousand Oaks, CA: Sage.

Ziegler, Mary. 2013. "Roe's Race: The Supreme Court, Population Control, and Reproductive Justice." *Yale Journal of Law & Feminism* 25 (1): article 2.

Zoelle, Diana Grace. 2000. *Globalizing Concern for Women's Human Rights: The Failure of the American Model*. New York: Springer.

INDEX

ABOUT THE AUTHOR

Zakiya Luna is Assistant Professor of Sociology and Feminist Studies at the University of California–Santa Barbara. She is coeditor of *Black Feminist Sociology: Perspectives and Praxis.* In her leisure time, she likes baking and learning to surf.

Printed and bound by CPI Group (UK) Ltd, Croydon, CR0 4YY

16/04/2025

14658443-0002